Taiwan Master Tung's Series

HIGHLIGHTS OF EFFECTIVE

POINTS SINCE 30 YEARS

IN CLINICAL CASES

An ancient Master Key that Resolves the Mystery That Western Medicine Cannot Solve

Karen Chang, my best friend, who change my life.

Copyright

Self-Publisher

About Author

Calvin Chien began his studies of Chinese Medicine in 1982, graduating with a Master's Degree in Acupuncture and Oriental Medicine (MAOM) in California. He has provided patients with the highest level of care since opening his own practice in 1997. Chien Acupuncture Clinic in Colorado Springs, CO continues to treat a variety of health concerns using traditional Chinese Medicine techniques including acupuncture, cupping, and herbal treatments. Calvin Chien diagnoses and treats clients who suffer from numerous health concerns. He is also the only practitioner and master in the fine art of "Master Tung's Acupuncture".

Dr. Calvin Chien's background includes:

Current president and primary acupuncturist of Chien Acupuncture clinic, Colorado Springs, CO

Current primary acupuncturist of Intensive Care Unit (ICU) in Penrose- St Francis Hospital, Colorado Springs, CO

Council Member of Council of Collge of Acupuncture and Oriental Medicine, CA

3rd generation acupuncturist that possesses a wealth of involvement and knowledge gleaned from generations of practicing acupuncturists.

having personal experience encompassing 30 years spent applying that knowledge, perfecting balance and acupuncture procedures combined with medicinal Chinese herbs, that have earned trust and respect from the community.

a vivid speaker and educator who advocating Tung's acupuncture and sharing clinical experience to physicians and acupuncturist in Taiwan and Japan.

The only practitioner and master in the fine art of "Master Tung's acupuncture" and "Master Tung's Palm Diagnosis"

For more Master Tung's information or seminar presentation, please contact information below:

calvin818@hotmail.com |
chienacupuncturecoloradospringsco.com
|Tel:719-799-3988| 4905
N Union #106, Colorado Springs, CO 80918

What are the actual Mr. Tung's extraordinary points in Taiwan? If there is an actual palmar diagnosis, only then there is the key!

Mr. Tung's extraordinary points, which are popular worldwide, have originated from clinical discoveries of five generations of ancestors and accumulation of experience. Therefore, these special acupuncture methods have been handed down from generation. Master Tung developed and unveiled this acupuncture method after coming to Taiwan, and nearly 400 thousand people have been diagnosed and treated using this method in the previous 30 years. His acupuncture method is different from the traditional ones. It has become a new school for the traditional science of acupuncture and moxibustion, but it is effective ineffably. It is highly praised by all acupuncturists. The advantage of Tung family's acupuncture is that it does not stick to any tonifying or reducing methods and needle manipulations. It helps identify the cause, recognize the acupuncture point, and then use the needle; it has a clear effect and immediately resolves old ailments!

This particular acupuncture must be matched with diagnosis to achieve a miraculous effect. For example, here is how Master Tung described himself at the 1962 world acupuncture conference: *"………Tung's diagnostic method is to check the color of both hands and arms first, and then look at the color of both sides of the face. Both of them can be combined to diagnose the disease and symptoms, and then acupoints are selected according to the channel. Its effectiveness is obvious!"* In other words, the patient does not need to describe their condition. A true disciple of Mr. Tung can diagnose the patient's disease as long as they see their palm. In addition, Master Tung also mentioned that when using this acupuncture method, it is necessary to indicate acupoints and use the correct diagnostic method through "word of mouth" and "personal instruction." Then, it will be easier to achieve success and reduce the suffering of patients. In this manner, we can learn the essence and crux of this ancestral acupuncture method.

The so-called acquisition of knowledge from the master means that there is a teacher who has clinical practice, helps the disciple in locating the acupoints, and teaches him about the "diagnosis" and "properties of the acupoints." It is just like making sushi. No one can learn the trick without entering the door. One cannot buy books and study it by oneself.

There are people who claim to be lecturers of Mr. Tung's extraordinary points and acupuncture in Taiwan; all of them themselves have bought books, plagiarized and inquired about different sources, and made irresponsible remarks because of which they make profit. All the "palm charts" and "acupoint charts" that are in circulation in the market are incorrect. They not only confuse those who actually want to learn but also embarrass Mr. Tung's family principles. There is even a second-generation descendant of Mr. Tung who had such a case where he caused infection during an operation, he was accused, and the California state government revoked his acupuncturist's license. What's ironic is that there are so many people follow and study Tung acupuncture. Isn't it weird? There is also another group of people who even perform Mr. Tung's acupuncture and moxibustion with "channel balance diagnosis," which is basically irrelevant as these methods are incompatible. The theories of Mr. Tung's extraordinary points have never been taught to anyone. Then, how come so many people call themselves teachers or students of Mr. Tung's extraordinary points? In particular, in the U.S., the so-called first generation of practitioners of Mr. Tung's extraordinary points is doubtful, let alone the later generations, who imitate the previous one. This is in line with the Chinese proverb which says that "A crooked stick will have a crooked shadow; it is virtually baffling."

How to identify whether a practitioner understands the actual theories of Mr. Tung's extraordinary points? The most direct and simple way is to extend your palm directly, and ask those who teach Tung's extraordinary points what kind of illness you have. In this way, you will distinguish whether he/she actually understands the theories. If you want to identify truly skilled people, just take our course and you will know. It is without tricks and is absolutely not phony. To put an end to these fraudulent, it is also specifically stated that Master Tung Chingchang did not have any students. Many lecturers, known as Master Tung's successors, are mostly his patients or military companies. It is wrong to claim that one is Mr. Tung's successor just because they had learned from Mr. Tung in the clinic. We also educate the public about the facts. Is it true that a shown skill may make one disappointed?

—Mr. Tung 's acupuncture and moxibustion, the third generation of authentic disciples

Calvin Nai Hsin Chien (O.MD, L. Ac)

CONTENTS

Common Painful Diseases

Generalized Pain

Formula One: Hegu (LI4)–Xuehai (SP10)
Acupuncture is performed. Insert the needles into the Hegu (LI4) and Xuehai (SP10), performing a reducing technique with strong stimulation. After achieving needle insertion sensation, leave the needles in place for 30 min.

Formula Two: Guanyuan (CV4)–Yinlingquan (SP9)
Acupuncture is performed. Insert the needles into the Guanyuan (CV4) and Yinlingquan (SP9), performing a uniform reinforcing-reducing technique. After achieving the needle insertion sensation, leave the needles in place for 30 min.

Case: Jackson, a 15-year-old American boy, caught a cold 3 weeks earlier. After treatment, all symptoms, except for sore throat, were relieved. Two weeks ago, he began to feel generalized pain, as if he was being pricked, with episodic exacerbation. The pain typically began from the knuckles and spread to his hands and feet. The pain lasted for 3–4 h each time, occurring 2–3 times each day. Generalized pain was diagnosed in this patient. After treatment with this method, pain disappeared and had not recurred at the 1-month follow-up.

This patient suffered from poor circulation of Qi and blood, which can cause pain. The pain is migratory and caused by exuberant wind. The Hegu (LI4) is a source (Yuan) point on a Yangming channel, which is abundant in Qi and blood. It can regulate the circulation of Qi and blood. This is accordance with the saying, regulate the blood first to regulate the Wind and the Wind will wane if the blood moves fluently. Therefore, the Hegu (LI4) and Xuehai (SP10) were selected for treatment in this case.

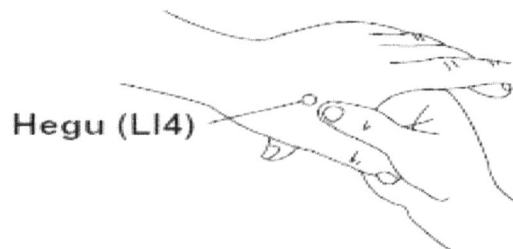

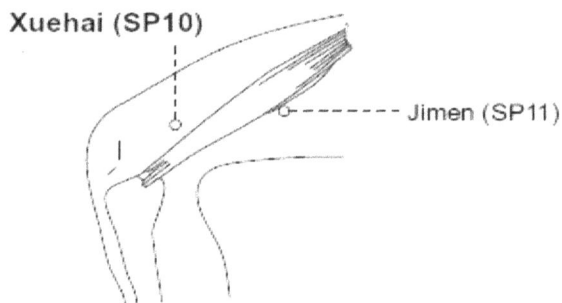

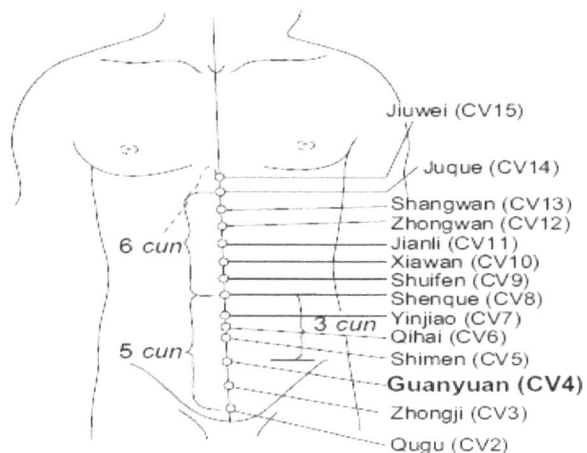

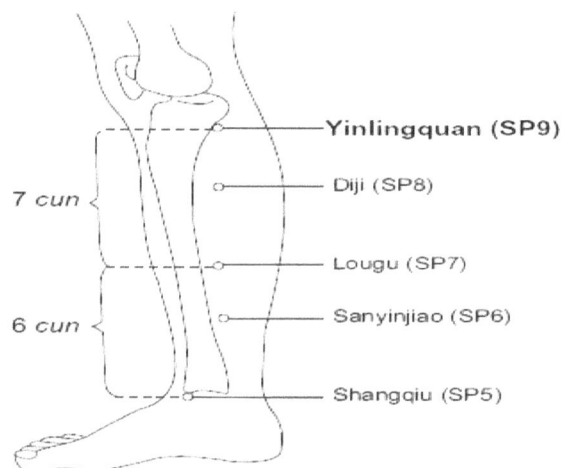

Eyebrow Bone Pain

Formula One: **Zhaohai (KI6)–Sanchasan (22.17)** (an extra Tong point located at the base between the little and ring finger)

Acupuncture is performed. Insert needles into the Zhaohai (KI6) and Sanchasan and leave them in place for 30 min.

Two patients suffering from eyebrow bone pain were treated with this method. In both patients, pain disappeared after two treatment sessions.

Formula Two: Lidui (ST45)–Cuanzhu (BL2)

Acupuncture is performed with the Zi Wu Liu Zhu (midnight–midday ebb flow) Nazi (hour prescription) technique. Insert a needle into the Lidui (ST45) at 8 a.m. (*Chen* hour) and then insert a needle into the Cuanzhu (BL2). Manipulate the needles once every 10 min, performing a reducing technique. Leave the needles in place for 60 min. After retaining the needles for 20 min, the left eyebrow bone pain should be halved. After removing the needles, the pain will disappear and the area around the eyebrow bone will be relaxed.

Case: Mr. Zhao, 29-year-old man, suffered from left eyebrow bone pain for 10 years, accompanied by dry mouth, desire for cold drinks, bloating, irritability, and dry stool. He had a furry, yellow tongue residue and a string-like rapid pulse. His head ached every morning from 7-to 9 a.m. (*Chen* hour). He was treated with this method and was cured after two sessions of treatment.

This patient suffered from too much heat invading the stomach, which can cause eyebrow bone pain from 7 to 9 a.m. (*Chen* hour). During this period, the stomach meridian is the main channel in the body. Qi and blood flow into the stomach meridian, causing stomach Qi to be exuberant. The stomach has the features of earth. As the Lidui (ST45) is a Jing-Well point on this channel, it has the features of gold and is the child of this channel. Therefore, we reduced the Lidui (ST45) during this period when the stomach meridian is excessive. The Nazi technique is a Zi Wu Liu Zhu technique in which five Shu points are selected in sequence according to time and their relationships to the mother–child using the theory of the five elements. This is in accordance to the saying, tonify the mother when suffering from deficiency and drain the child when suffering from excess.

Eyebrow Bone Pain Points

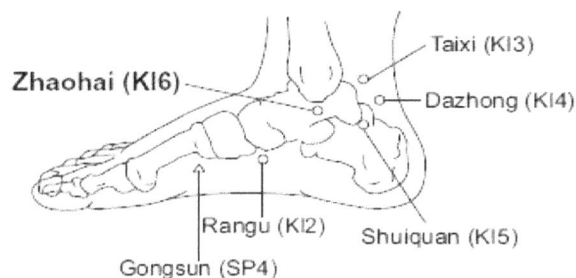

Zhaohai (KI6), Taixi (KI3), Dazhong (KI4), Rangu (KI2), Shuiquan (KI5), Gongsun (SP4)

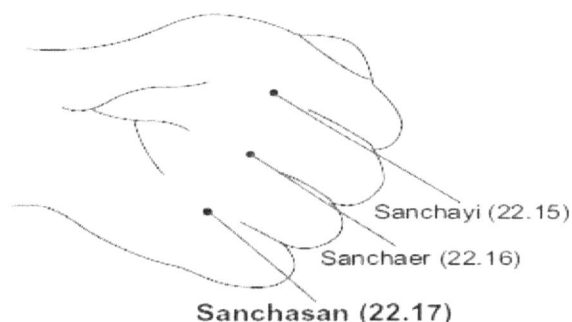

Sanchayi (22.15), Sanchaer (22.16), Sanchasan (22.17)

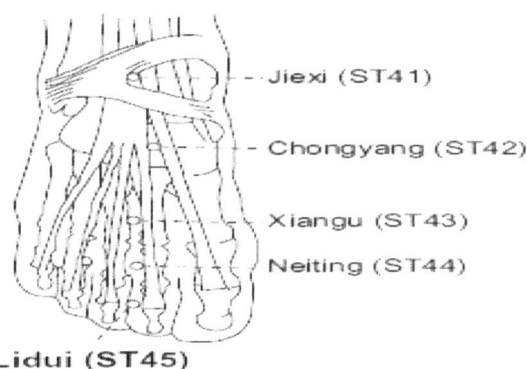

Jiexi (ST41), Chongyang (ST42), Xiangu (ST43), Neiting (ST44), Lidui (ST45)

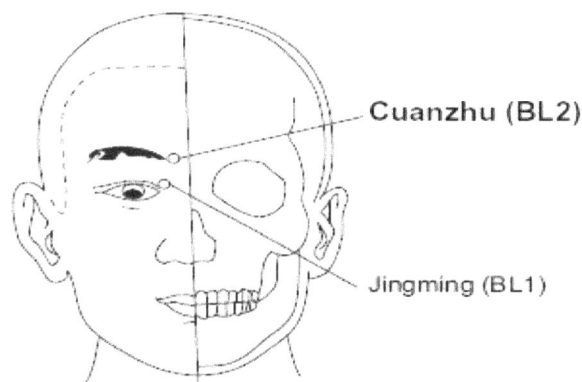

Cuanzhu (BL2), Jingming (BL1)

Neck and Shoulder Pain

Neck and Shoulder Pain

Formula One: Wangu (SI4)–Shenmen (HT7)

Acupuncture is performed. During the episode of pain (from Wu to Wei hour), insert a needle into the Wangu (SI4), performing a reducing technique. Then insert another needle into the Shenmen (HT7), performing a reinforcing technique. Leave the needles in place for 20 min.

After one session of treatment with this method, neck and shoulder pain will disappear.

Formula Two: Ashi point–Shousanli (LI10)

Case: Mr. Li, a 45-year-old American man, suffered from his neck and shoulder pain on the left side and had been unable to move this area for 5–10 days. He underwent electro-acupuncture at a Traditional Chinese Medicine (TCM) clinic, but it did not help. Examination revealed that the left edge of the trapezius muscle, from Fengchi (GB20) to Jianzhongshu (SI15), was stiff and accompanied by tenderness. Tenderness also occurred at the left Shousanli (LI10). This syndrome is termed stiff neck and can be cured by two sessions of treatment with this method.

This patient suffered from a block in the channels and poor circulation of Qi and blood. Acupuncture or acupressure could be effective. As the saying goes, a specific syndrome can be cured by treatment of related channels. The Shousanli (LI10) is present on the large intestine channel, which is a Yangming channel, and is abundant in Qi and blood. A syndrome of stagnation of Qi and blood can cause symptoms, such as tenderness of the area where the Yangming channels pass. Performing acupuncture on this channel can cure this syndrome.

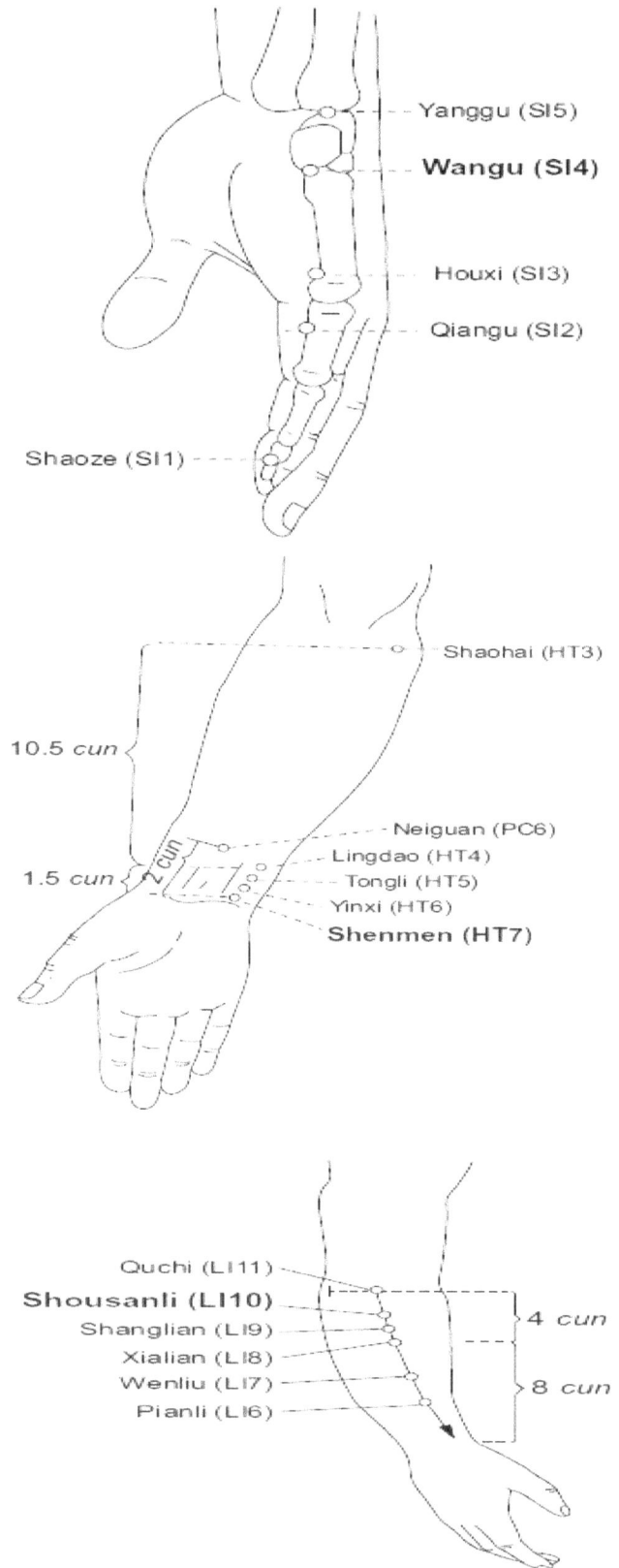

Shoulder Pain

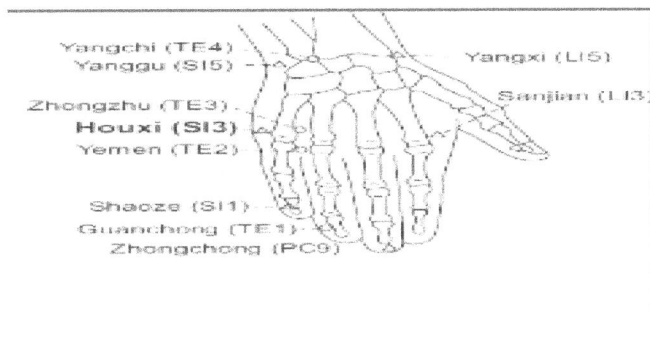

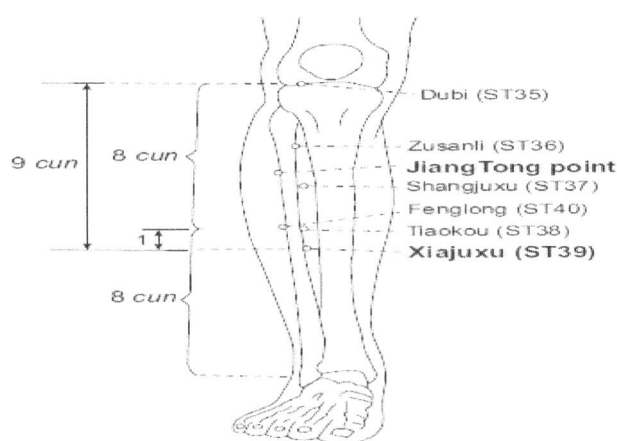

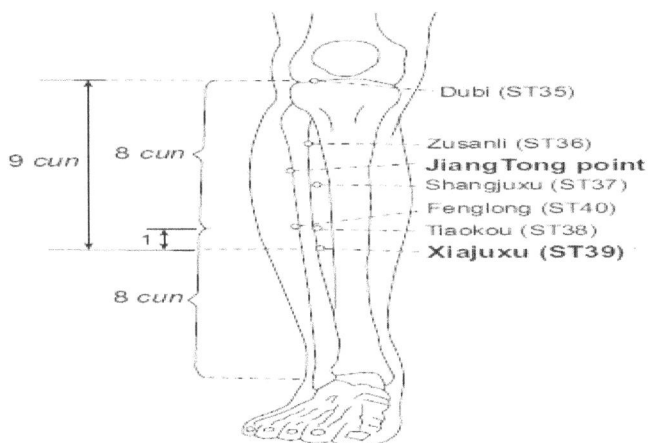

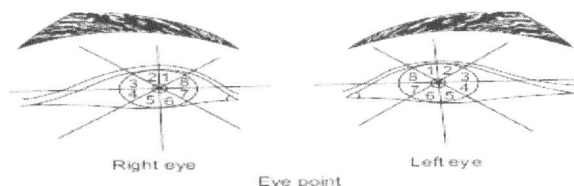

Treatment of shoulder pain with paired acupoints was recorded by Gao Wu in the Ming Dynasty (1368–1644 A.D.) in his book Zhenjiu Juying: "If the shoulder is swollen and has a dragging sensation, the Guanyuan (CV4) should be selected. After three sessions of treatment with moxibustion at this point, the discomfort will wane. If moxibustion is performed on Dadun (LR1), discomfort will disappear after seven sessions of treatment." Gao Wu believed that moxibustion on the Guanyuan (CV4) and Dadun (LR1) is effective in treating swollen and painful shoulders.

Formula One: Houxi (SI3)–Xiajuxu (ST39)

Acupuncture is performed. Insert a needle into the Houxi (SI3) at 0.5–1 *cun* deep. The needle can penetrate through the Laogong (PC8). Insert another needle into the Xiajuxu (ST39) at 1–1.5 *cun* deep, performing a reducing technique by lifting and thrusting of the needle. Leave the needle in place for 20 min. Ask the patient to move the affected shoulder. Usually, the first treatment is effective, i.e., efficacy rate is 97%.

Case: Steven, a 41-year-old American man, suffered from shoulder pain and could not raise his arm for 1 month. The symptoms became worse because of cold weather and overwork. He was treated at another clinic, but the treatment was not effective. After two sessions of treatment at our clinic, his symptoms disappeared.

Formula Two: Jiantong–Shangjiaoqu (Eye point)

Case: Ms. Li, a 40-year-old Taiwanese woman suffered from periarthritis of the left shoulder for 10 months. She had trouble with intorsion, abduction, lifting, and rear extension using her upper left extremity. After one session of treatment with acupuncture on these two points, her symptoms disappeared.

When using the Jiantong point to treat periarthritis of the shoulder, the key is to regulate the neural system, which is the supreme system regulating the body's adaptation to the environment.

The Jiantong point: Located 2 *cun* under the Zusanli (ST36) and 1 *cun* outside of it.

Shangjiaoqu (eye point): Located according to Jingshan Peng's theory, which differs from the theory of Dong eye points.

Eye point

Right eye   Left eye

1. Fei Dachang (Lung and Large Intestine)
2. Shen Pangguang (Kidney and Bladder)
3. **Shangjiao (Upper Energizer)**
4. Gandan (Liver and Gallbladder)
5. Zhongjiao (Middle Energizer)
6. Xin Xiaochang (Heart and Small Intestine)
7. Piwei (Spleen and Stomach)
8. Xiajiao (Lower Energizer)

Scapular Region Pain

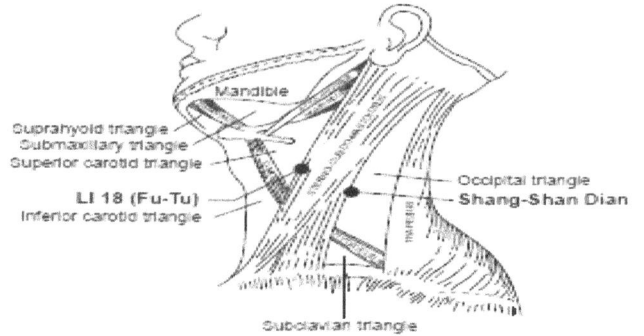

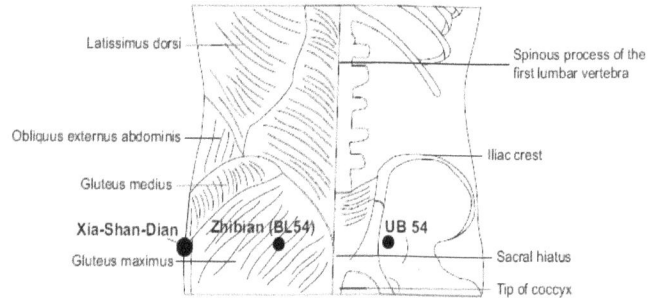

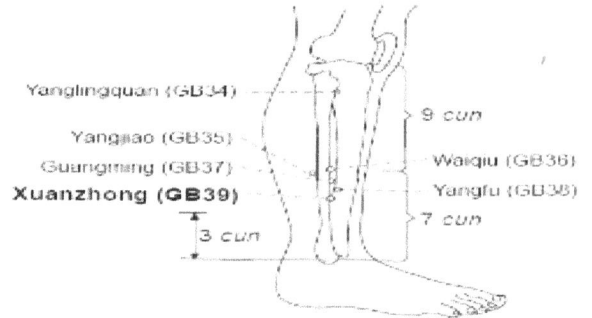

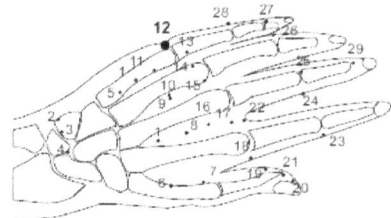

Formula One: Shangshandian–Xiashandian

Shangshandian: An extra point located at the outer edge of the sternocleidomastoid.

Xiashandian: An extra point located 6 *cun* outside the S2 vertebrae. It is also located 3 *cun* outside the Zhibian (BL54). The Xiashandian, Zhibian (BL54), and Huantiao (GB30), which are located at the edge of the gluteus medius muscle, gluteus minimus, and greater sciatic notch, respectively, form a triangle.

We have treated 265 cases of scapular region pain using this method. Treatment was effective in all cases, i.e., the efficacy rate was 100%.

This pair of points can also be effective for treating other diseases. If these points are used well, a great benefit can be obtained.

Formula Two: Xuanzhong (GB39)–Jizhu (Hand point)

Jizhu (Hand point): To find this point, ask the patient to make a fist. This point is near the base joint of the little finger and is located at the dorso–ventral boundary of the hand.

Acupuncture manipulation: Insert the needle perpendicularly 3 *fen* deep. The tip of the needle should touch the bone.

This pair of points can be used for treating interspinous ligament sprain and latissimus dorsi pain. Treatment is immediately effective

Scapular Region Pain

Mandible
Suprahyoid triangle
Submaxillary triangle
Superior carotid triangle
LI 18 (Fu-Tu)
Inferior carotid triangle
Occipital triangle
Shang-Shan Dian
Subclavian triangle

Latissimus dorsi
Spinous process of the first lumbar vertebra
Obliquus externus abdominis
Iliac crest
Gluteus medius
Xia-Shan-Dian   Zhibian (BL54)   UB 54
Gluteus maximus
Sacral hiatus
Tip of coccyx

Yanglingquan (GB34)
Yangjiao (GB35)
Guangming (GB37)
Xuanzhong (GB39)
9 cun
Waiqiu (GB36)
Yangfu (GB38)
7 cun
3 cun

1. Yaotui (Lower back and leg)
2. Jiakang (Hyperthyreosis)
3. Zhixue (Stop bleeding)
4. Shengya (Raise blood pressure)
5. Nvfu
6. Diankuang Gaoxueya (Mania and high blood pressure)
7. Shuimian (Sleep)
8. Yunche (Motion sickness)
9. Fuxie (Diarrhea)
10. Xiongshang (Chest injury)
11. Jianshang (Shoulder injury)
12. Jizhu (Spine)
13. Zuogu Shenjing (Sciatic nerve)
14. Bidian (Nose)
15. Yanhou (Throat)
16. Luolingwu
17. Jingxiang (Neck)
18. Jiandian (Shoulder)
19. Yandian (Eye)
20. Shenyan Shuizhong (Nephretis and swelling)
21. Yemang (Night blindness)
22. Tuire (Reduce fever)
23. Qiantou (Forehead)
24. Touding (Top of head)
25. Ouzhang (Vomit and bloating)
26. Piantou (Sides of head)
27. Houtong (Sore throat)
28. Houtou (Back of head)
29. Eni (Hiccup)

Chest and Abdominal Pain

Formula One: Zusanli (ST36)–Zhiyang (GV9)

We have used this method to treat chest and abdominal pain in 200 cases. It was effective in 195 cases, i.e., the total efficacy rate was 97.55%.

Each organ is related to some points on the skin. When these points are stimulated because of diseases of the related organ, it causes pain. If untreated, this pain can be a vicious stimulation on the cerebral cortex. Abdominal pain is caused by a disorder of the visceral autonomic nervous system and conducted by sensory nerves in the abdomen. Acupuncture stimulates the skin, balancing the distribution of greater splanchnic nerves and transmitting signals to the cerebral cortex to produce positive effect.

Chest and Abdomen Pain

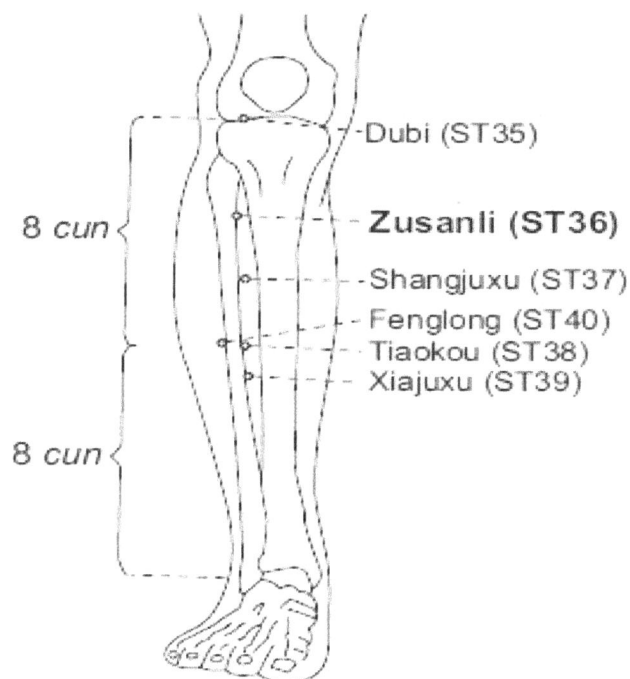

8 cun

Dubi (ST35)
Zusanli (ST36)
Shangjuxu (ST37)
Fenglong (ST40)
Tiaokou (ST38)
Xiajuxu (ST39)

8 cun

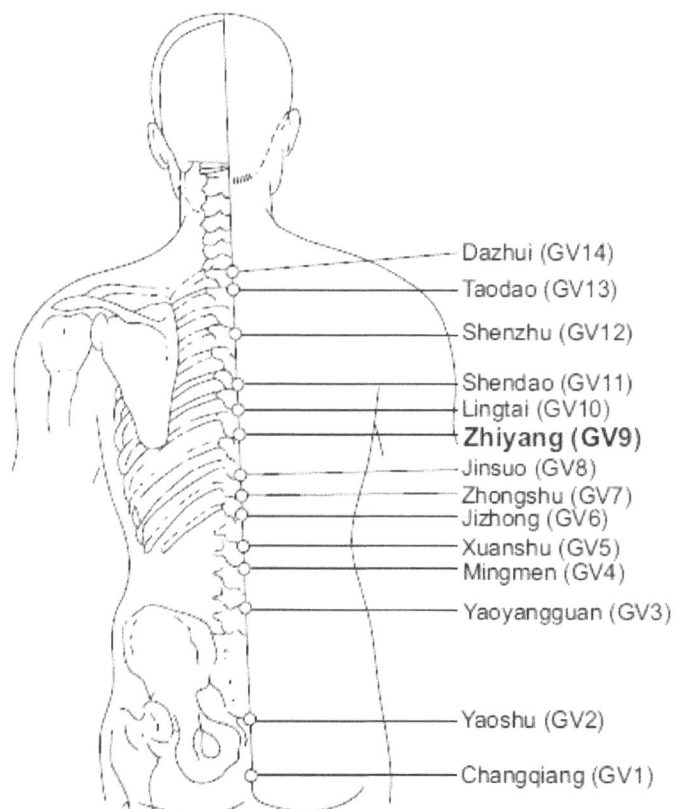

Dazhui (GV14)
Taodao (GV13)
Shenzhu (GV12)
Shendao (GV11)
Lingtai (GV10)
Zhiyang (GV9)
Jinsuo (GV8)
Zhongshu (GV7)
Jizhong (GV6)
Xuanshu (GV5)
Mingmen (GV4)
Yaoyangguan (GV3)
Yaoshu (GV2)
Changqiang (GV1)

Back Pain
Formula One: Jinmen (BL63)–Zhongzhu (TE3)

Dong-Qi acupuncture is performed. Leave the needles in place for 30 min. In practice, we often meet patients who complain of back pain, specifically, thoracic segment pain. Usually, these patients have already been treated with western medicine. Often, in such patients no cause or pathologic sign was found and no diagnosis could be confirmed. Thus, there was no effective treatment in western medicine. From the perspective of traditional Chinese medicine, however, such patients can be treated with acupuncture, which tends to be effective.

The Jinmen (BL63) is a distal point. The Zhongzhu (TE3) is the Shu-Stream point of the Triple Energizer channel. The triple energizers are responsible for Qi transformation and can warm muscles and enrich the skin. Acupuncture on the Zhongzhu (TE3) can invigorate the Governor vessel, motivate Yang Qi, and unblock channels to help stop pain. This pair of points, whose effectiveness has been recognized in practice, is for reference.

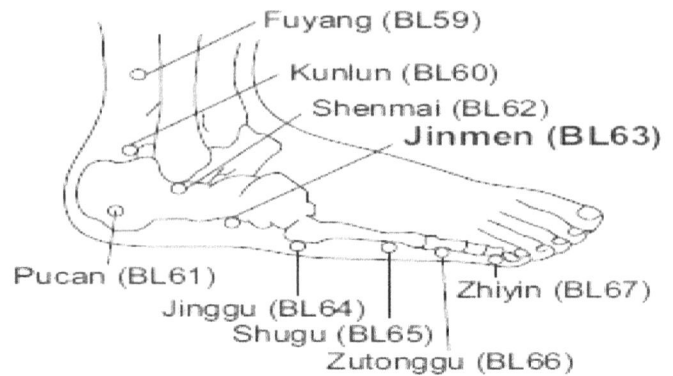

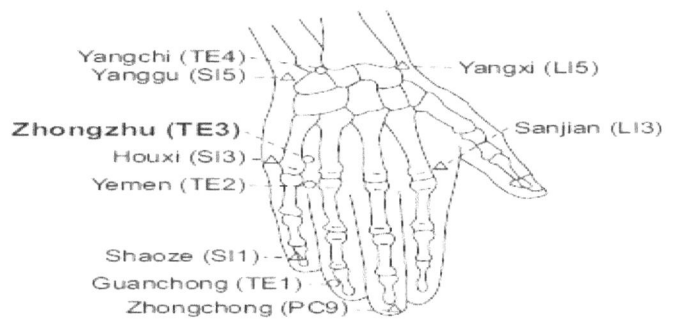

Formula Two: Shenguan (77.18)–Erjiaoming (11.12)

This pair of points is Dong's "miraculous formula." They are flexibly used by many practitioners and are extremely effective. Besides pain caused by spinal curvature, they can be used for treating lower back pain.

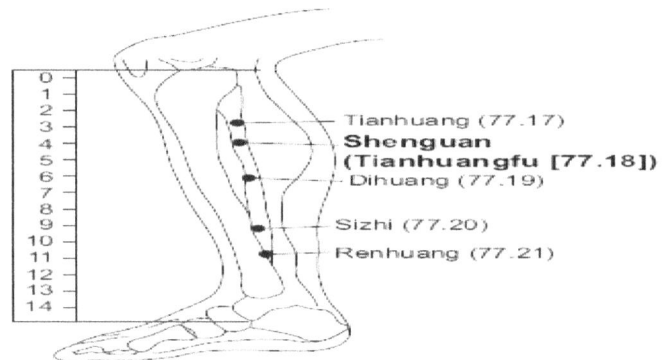

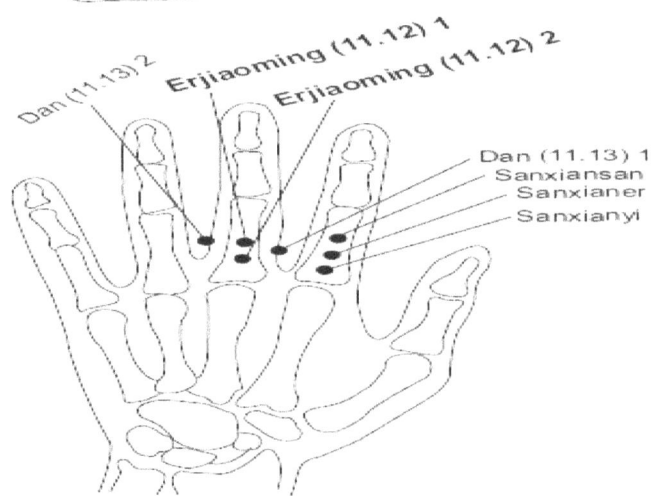

Back Pain

Elbow Pain

Formula One: Yanglingquan (GB34)–Dubi (ST35)

Perform acupuncture using a reducing technique with twisting needles. Leave the needles in place for 30 min.

Case: Mr. Guan, aged 42 years, suffered from right elbow pain for 3 months and had a problem with the flexion and extension function. Examination showed tenderness of the right lateral epicondyle of the humerus. The affected area was located between the hand Shaoyang and Yangming channels. Channels with the same name were selected. "When diseases are in the upper part of the body, channels and points in the lower part of the body are selected." Thus, the foot Shaoyang and Yangming channels were selected. After five sessions of treatment with this method, the flexion and extension function of the elbow was restored.

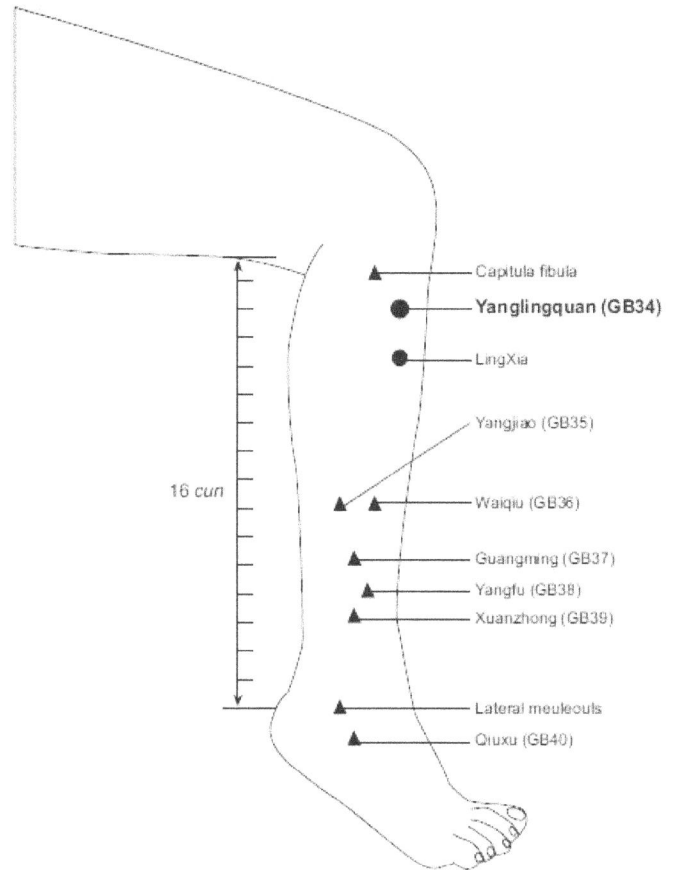

16 cun

- Capitula fibula
- **Yanglingquan (GB34)**
- LingXia
- Yangjiao (GB35)
- Waiqiu (GB36)
- Guangming (GB37)
- Yangfu (GB38)
- Xuanzhong (GB39)
- Lateral meuleouls
- Qiuxu (GB40)

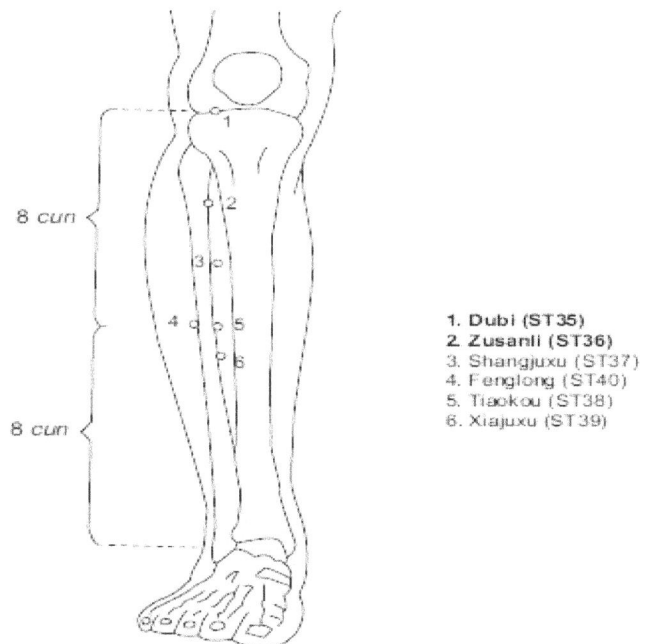

8 cun

8 cun

1. **Dubi (ST35)**
2. **Zusanli (ST36)**
3. Shangjuxu (ST37)
4. Fenglong (ST40)
5. Tiaokou (ST38)
6. Xiajuxu (ST39)

Rib Pain

Formula One: Yuji (LU10)–Weizhong (BL40)

Acupuncture is performed. Insert needles into the affected side, performing a reducing technique. Leave the needles in place for 30 min.

This method is for reference. We used it to effectively treat rib pain caused by injury.

Formula Two: Neiguan (PC6)–Taichong (LR3)

Acupuncture is performed. Insert needles perpendicularly 1 *cun* deep, performing a reinforcing or reducing technique. Do not twist the needles. Leave the needles in place for 20 min.

For patients who commonly suffer from rib pain because of bad mood, one session of this treatment can stop the pain.

Rib Pain

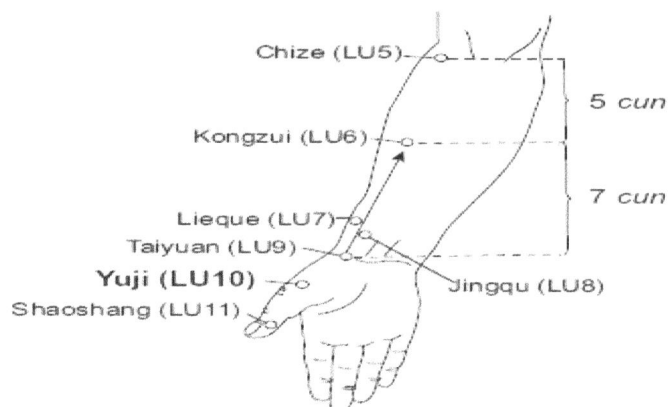

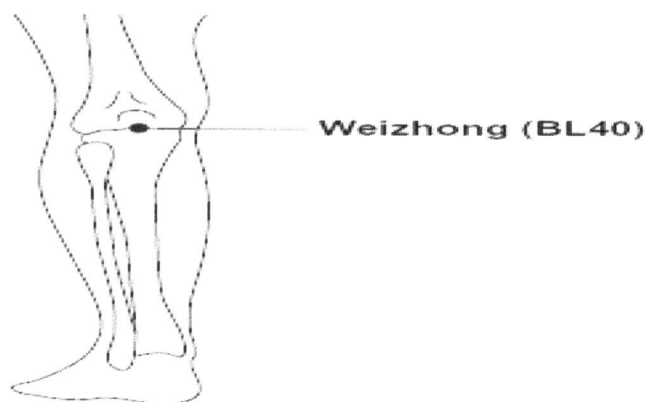

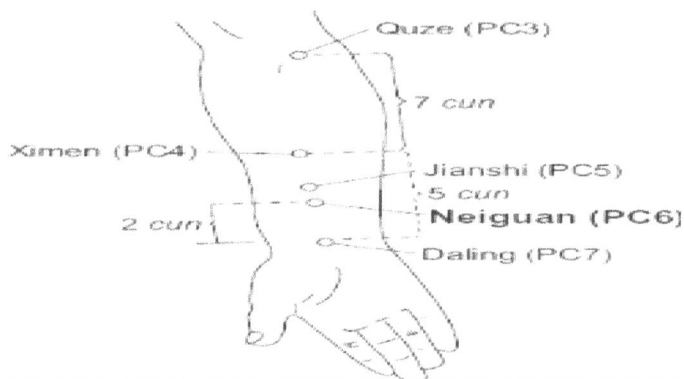

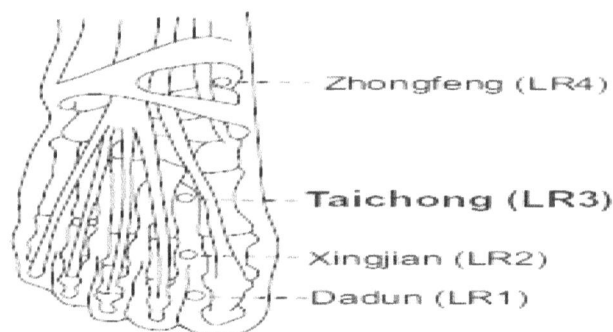

Lower Back Pain

Formula One: Ashi point–Kunlun (BL60)

Acupuncture is performed. Select the tenderness point as the Ashi point on the right hand and the Kunlun (BL60) on the left hand. Perform a reducing technique while twisting and twirling the needle. Simultaneously, ask the patient to turn their waist. After 3 min, the pain will be eased. Then, leave the needles for 10 more min. After removing the needles, massage the waist to relax the muscles.

Case: Li, a 35-year-old Singaporean man, experienced lower back pain after bearing a load and spraining his back. He had problems with turning, flexion, and extension. On examination, obvious tenderness at the Dachangshu (BL25) was observed. He had a thin, furry tongue residue and a string-like tight pulse. Lower back pain was diagnosed in the patient and was cured after one session of treatment with this method.

Formula Two: Houxi (SI3)–Shuigou (GV26)

Acupuncture on these points is performed to treat lower back pain. Most patients (>90%) will experience immediate effectiveness. In practice, these points are selected for treating lower back pain without syndromic differentiation. Practitioners can use this method to ease pain immediately, and subsequently perform acupuncture according to a more specific diagnosis.

Lower Back Pain

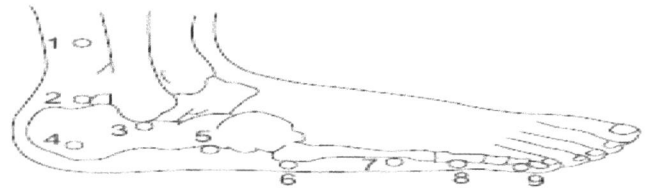

1. Fuyang (BL59)
2. **Kunlun (BL60)**
3. Shenmai (BL62)
4. Pucan (BL61)
5. Jinmen (BL63)
6. Jinggu (BL64)
7. Shugu (BL65)
8. Zutonggu (BL66)
9. Zhiyin (BL67)

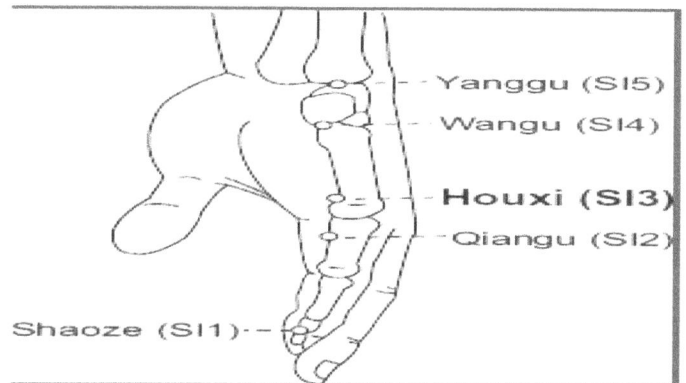

Yanggu (SI5)
Wangu (SI4)
Houxi (SI3)
Qiangu (SI2)
Shaoze (SI1)

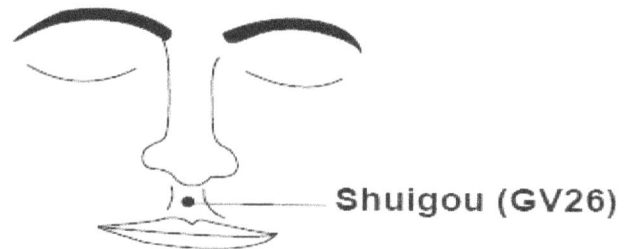

Shuigou (GV26)

Lower Back and Leg Pain

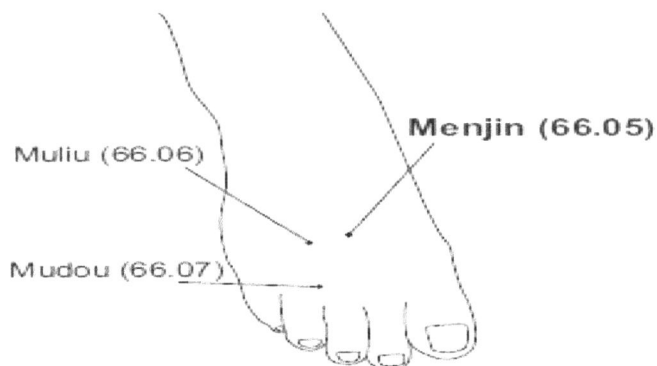

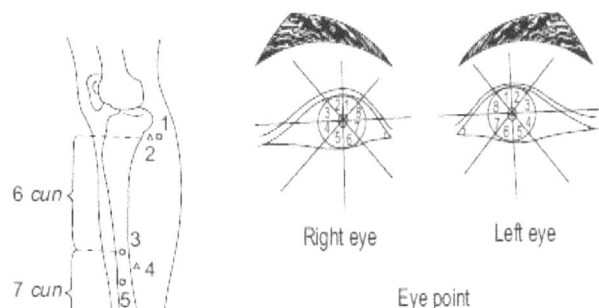

Formula One: Menjin (66.05)–Zhongdu (LR6)

It is our desire to publicize this pair of antalgic points without any specific needle technique. Select points on the affected side. It is possible to realize a remarkable effect using the Dong-Qi technique. However, the cause of pain should be confirmed. If pain is caused by compression of the sciatic nerve, other acupoints should be selected.

Lower back and leg pain are a common symptom. It is caused by improper posture during exercise, overload, or chronic strain on the soft tissue. All of these problems can cause blockage of channels. Besides acupuncture, which has an immediate effect, manipulation can be very effective.

Formula Two: Xiajiaoqu (Eye point)–Fuliu (KI7)

This pair of points is for reference. They can be used for treating lower back and leg pain. The pain will stop after two sessions of treatment. A breath reducing technique should be used. Dong's control needling method may also be used.

Lower Back and Leg Pain

Muliu (66.06)
Menjin (66.05)
Mudou (66.07)

6 cun
7 cun

Right eye   Left eye

Eye point

1. Fei Dachang (Lung and Large Intestine)
2. Shen Pangguang (Kidney and Bladder)
3. Shangjiao (Upper Energizer)
4. Gandan (Liver and Gallbladder)
5. Zhongjiao (Middle Energizer)
6. Xin Xiaochang (Heart and Small Intestine)
7. Piwei (Spleen and Stomach)
8. Xiajiao (Lower Energizer)

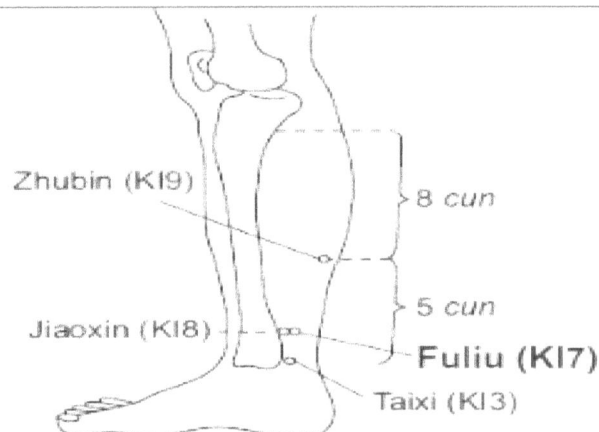

1. Xiguan (LR7)
2. Yinlingquan (SP9)
3. Zhongdu (LR6)
4. Lougu (SP7)
5. Ligou (LR5)

Zhubin (KI9)
8 cun
5 cun
Jiaoxin (KI8)
Fuliu (KI7)
Taixi (KI3)

Sacrococcygeal Region Pain
Formula One: Baihui (GV20)–Didian (Hand point)

Acupuncture is performed, without any specific needle technique. Sacrococcygeal region pain is mostly caused by fall and injury, which causes the channels to be blocked. Qi and blood cannot circulate freely, and this obstruction causes pain.

Case: Ms. Wang, a 60-year-old woman suffered from sacrococcygeal region pain and stayed in bed for 3 days. She could not turn around, sit, or stand. The pain worsened when straining during bowel movements. On examination, X-ray showed no abnormity. The result of the knee-jerk test was positive. After treatment for 3–5 min, the pain disappeared and did not recur.

Sacrococcygeal Region Pain

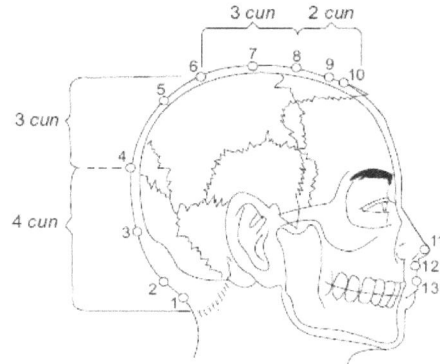

1. Yamen (GV15)
2. Fengfu (GV16)
3. Naohu (GV17)
4. Qiangjian (GV18)
5. Houding (GV19)
6. **Baihui (GV20)**
7. Qianding (GV21)
8. Xinhui (GV22)
9. Shangxing (GV23)
10. Shenting (GV24)
11. Suliao (GV25)
12. Shuigou (GV26)
13. Duiduan (GV27)

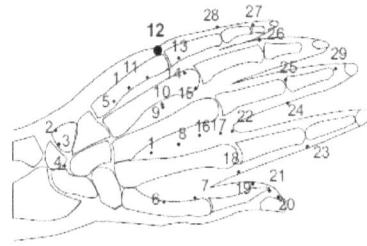

1. Yaotui (Lower back and leg)
2. Jiakang (Hyperthyreosis)
3. Zhixue (Stop bleeding)
4. Shengya (Raise blood pressure)
5. Nvfu
6. Diankuang Gaoxueya (Mania and high blood pressure)
7. Shuimian (Sleep)
8. Yunche (Motion sickness)
9. Fuxie (Diarrhea)
10. Xiongshang (Chest injury)
11. Jianshang (Shoulder injury)
12. **Jizhu (Spine)**
13. Zuogu Shenjing (Sciatic nerve)
14. Bidian (Nose)
15. Yanhou (Throat)
16. Luolingwu
17. Jingxiang (Neck)
18. Jiandian (Shoulder)
19. Yandian (Eye)
20. Shenyan Shuizhong (Nephretis and swelling)
21. Yemang (Night blindness)
22. Tuire (Reduce fever)
23. Qiantou (Forehead)
24. Touding (Top of head)
25. Ouzhang (Vomit and bloating)
26. Piantou (Sides of head)
27. Houtong (Sore throat)
28. Houtou (Back of head)
29. Eni (Hiccup)
30. **Didian**

Lower Extremity Pain

Formula One: Gandanqu (Eye point)–Xiajiaoqu (Eye point)

Acupuncture on the eye point is performed. The Gandanqu and Xiajiaoqu are selected. Leave the needle in place for 20 min. Lower extremity pain should stop after one session of treatment with this method.

Chinese eye acupuncture was developed by Peng and was popularized in mainland China. The points and treatment differ from those of Dong. Practitioners who were taught by their masters can use these eye points flexibly to treat stroke and miscellaneous diseases. This is also a miraculous treatment. We would like to publicize this technique and discuss it with colleagues to promote development of Taiwanese acupuncture.

Lower Extremity Pain

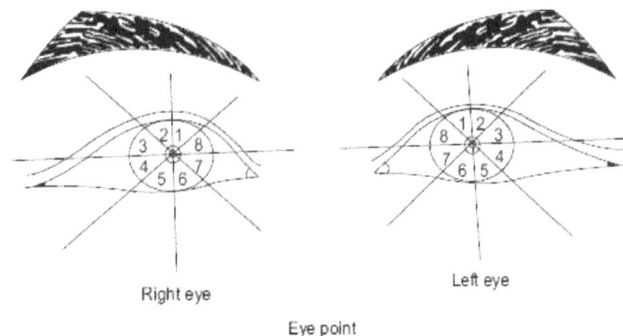

Right eye   Left eye

Eye point

1. Fei Dachang (Lung and Large Intestine)
2. Shen Pangguang (Kidney and Bladder)
3. Shangjiao (Upper Energizer)
4. **Gandan (Liver and Gallbladder)**
5. Zhongjiao (Middle Energizer)
6. Xin Xiaochang (Heart and Small Intestine)
7. Piwei (Spleen and Stomach)
8. **Xiajiao (Lower Energizer)**

Knee Pain

Formula One: Shenqu, Danqu (Navel point)–Xixue (Face point)

Acupuncture is performed. Insert the needles perpendicularly, performing a uniform reinforcing-reducing technique.

Xixue (Face point): It is located on the line between the earlobe and angle of the mandible and one-third of the distance from the angle of the mandible to the earlobe.

Select this pair of points and leave the needles in place for 15 min once per day.

1. Knee pain, which worsens when walking up and down stairs or squatting. The pain is obvious when standing up after sitting for a long time. The knee may be red and swollen.

2. The pain worsens on rainy days. Most patients with this symptom are middle-aged.

3. X-ray indicates osteophytes in the knee joints.

Formula Two: Xinxi (11.09)–Xuanzhong (GB39)

The Xinxi (11.09) is located on the sides of the middle finger, at the middle point between the fingertip and base joint.

Acupuncture is performed, without any specific needle technique. Patients with acute pain are usually cured after one session of treatment. We publicize this effective pair of points for reference.

KneePain

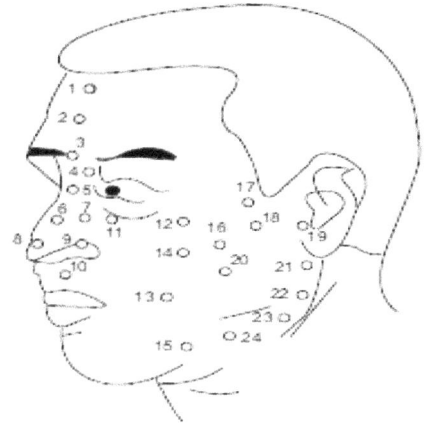

1. Toumian (Head and Face)
2. Yanhou (Throat)
3. Feixue (Lung)
4. Yingru (Breast)
5. Xinxue (Heart)
6. Ganxue (Liver)
7. Danxue (Gallbladder)
8. Pixue (Spleen)
9. Weixue (Stomach)
10. Pangguang (Bladder)
11. Xiaochang (Small Intestine)
12. Jianxue (Shoulder)
13. Guli (Groin)
14. Dachang (Large Intestine)
15. Zuxue (Foot)
16. Shenxue (Kidney)
17. Bixue (Arm)
18. Shouxue (Hand)
19. Beixue (Back)
20. Qixue (Navel)
21. Guxue (Thigh)
22. **Xixue (Knee)**
23. Xibing (Patella)
24. Jingxue (Shin)

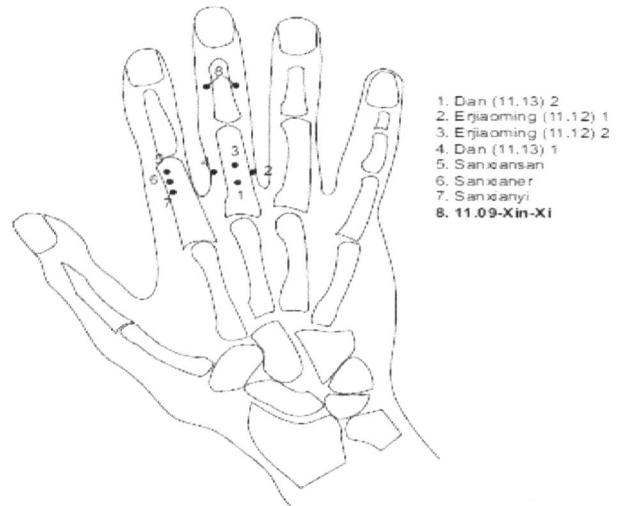

1. Dan (11.13) 2
2. Erjiaoming (11.12) 1
3. Erjiaoming (11.12) 2
4. Dan (11.13) 1
5. Sanxiansan
6. Sanxianer
7. Sanxianyi
8. **11.09-Xin-Xi**

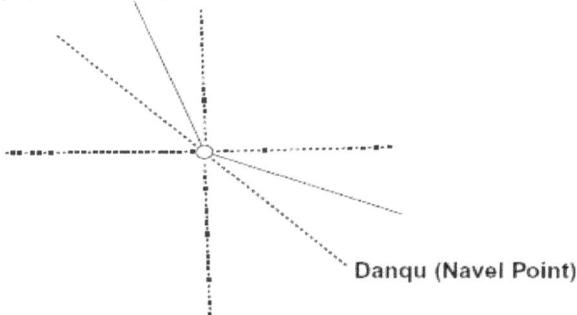

Shenqu (Navel Point)

Danqu (Navel Point)

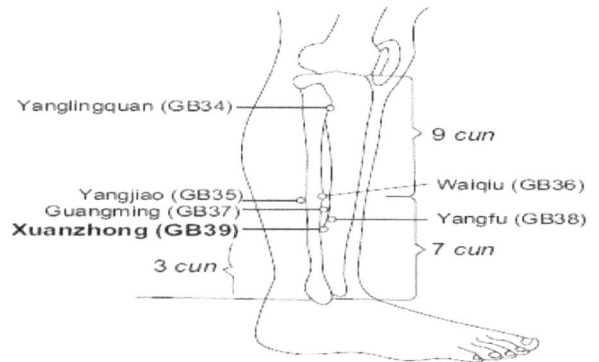

Yanglingquan (GB34)

9 cun

Yangjiao (GB35)
Guangming (GB37)
Xuanzhong (GB39)

Waiqiu (GB36)

Yangfu (GB38)

7 cun

3 cun

Ankle and Toe Pain

Formula One: Hegu (LI4)–Kunlun (BL60)

Needles measuring 0.22 × 40 mm are used. Acupuncture is performed. Insert a needle perpendicularly into the Hegu (LI4) on the affected side. Insert another needle downward obliquely into the Kunlun (BL60) on the same side. After achieving needle insertion sensation, leave the needles in place for 10 min. Next, perform the Dong-Qi technique and move the affected foot for 5 min. Remove the needles when the pain disappears. This technique can be very effective.

Formula Two: Xiajiaoqu (Eye point)

This point is used as an assistant point.

Ankle and Toe Pain

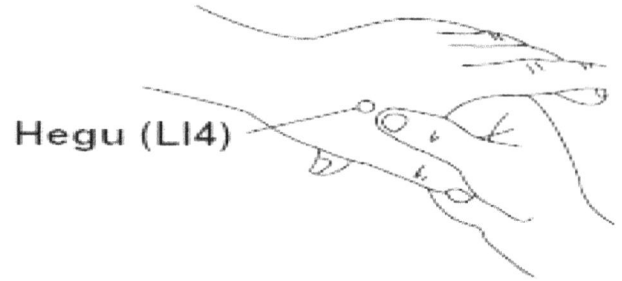

Hegu (LI4)

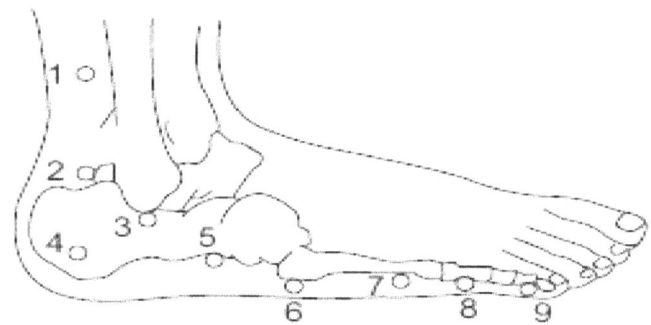

1. Fuyang (BL59)
2. **Kunlun (BL60)**
3. Shenmai (BL62)
4. Pucan (BL61)
5. Jinmen (BL63)
6. Jinggu (BL64)
7. Shugu (BL65)
8. Zutonggu (BL66)
9. Zhiyin (BL67)

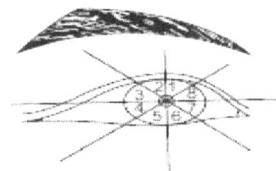

Right eye

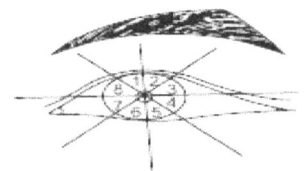

Left eye

Eye point

1. Fei Dachang (Lung and Large Intestine)
2. Shen Pangguang (Kidney and Bladder)
3. Shangjiao (Upper Energizer)
4. Gandan (Liver and Gallbladder)
5. Zhongjiao (Middle Energizer)
6. Xin Xiaochang (Heart and Small Intestine)
7. Piwei (Spleen and Stomach)
8. **Xiajiao (Lower Energizer)**

Heel Pain

Treatment for heel pain is the same as that for ankle and toe pain. It was first reported by Gao Wu in the Ming Dynasty (1368–1644 A.D.) in Zhenjiu Juying: "Diseases beneath the ankle should be treated with moxibustion on the Zhaohai (KI6). If it is accompanied with moxibustion on the Shenmai (BL62), the diseases can be completely cured." In his opinion, heel pain should be treated using the Zhaohai (KI6) and Shenmai (BL62) at both sides of the ankle.

Formula One: Hegu (LI4)–Kunlun (BL60)

Acupuncture is performed. Select points on the affected side. Heel pain is mostly caused by kidney deficiency and insufficiency of essence and blood. Kidney deficiency can cause poor circulation of Qi and blood, inducing nodes generated under the feet. The syndrome is deficiency in origin and excess in superficiality. Thus, a reducing technique should be performed.

Case: Calvin, a 52-year-old man, suffered from pain on the outer edge of his right heel for more than half a year. The pain was particularly severe in the morning when getting up. It felt as if his heel was being poked. He took anti-inflammatory medication and cortisone. However, the medications were ineffective. He was treated with this pair of points combined with herbal medicine. The pain stopped after two sessions of treatment.

Heel Pain

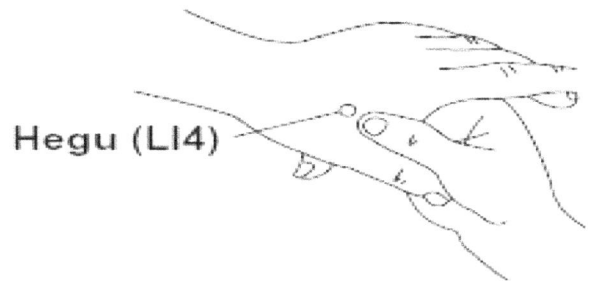

Hegu (LI4)

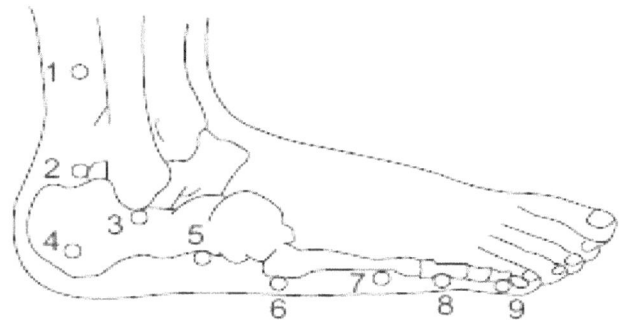

1. Fuyang (BL59)
2. **Kunlun (BL60)**
3. Shenmai (BL62)
4. Pucan (BL61)
5. Jinmen (BL63)
6. Jinggu (BL64)
7. Shugu (BL65)
8. Zutonggu (BL66)
9. Zhiyin (BL67)

Incision Pain

Formula One: Ashi point–Shenmen (Ear point)

Shenmen (Ear point): It is located at the lateral third of the triangular fossa, near the superior crus of the antihelix.

Acupuncture is performed. We have treated incision pain using this method in 50 cases. It was clearly effective in 45 cases, effective in 2 cases, and ineffective in 3 cases. The total efficacy rate was 94%.

Incision Pain

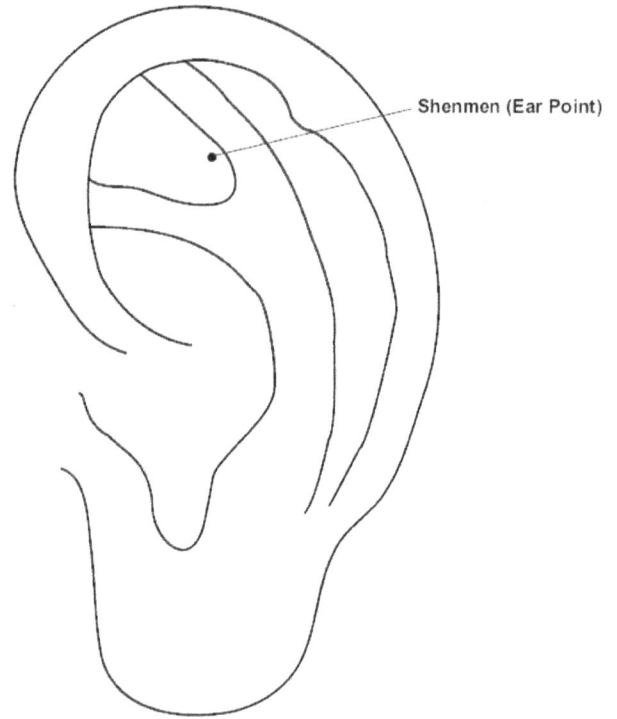

Shenmen (Ear Point)

Pain and Cold Feeling in the Knee

Pain and Cold Feeling in the Knee

Formula One: Dubi (ST35)–Zusanli (ST36)

Acupuncture is performed. First, insert needles into the Dubi (ST35) and Zusanli (ST36) on the right side, performing a warm reinforcing technique. Lift and thrust the needles approximately 10 times. The patient will feel warmth at the right knee. The sensation may spread to the right foot dorsum. Next, perform the same technique on the left side.

Case: We used this method to treat an alpinist aged 42 years. He had felt pain and a cold feeling in both knees for 10 days, and it was more severe on the right side. He experienced discomfort while walking. He had no problem consuming cold food or drinks. We diagnosed him with pain and cold feeling in knee and treated him with this method. After two sessions of treatment, the symptoms disappeared.

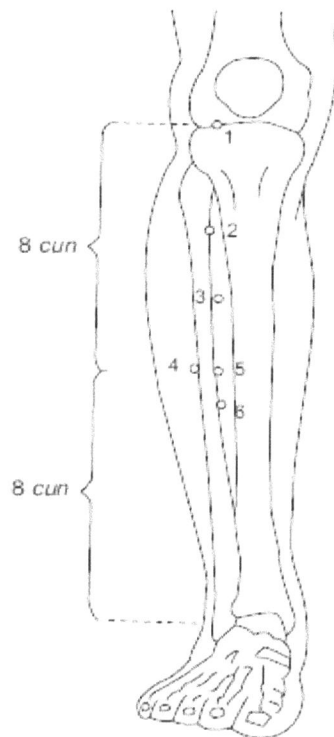

8 cun

8 cun

1. Dubi (ST35)
2. Zusanli (ST36)
3. Shangjuxu (ST37)
4. Fenglong (ST40)
5. Tiaokou (ST38)
6. Xiajuxu (ST39)

Chapter Two

Injury
Stiff Neck

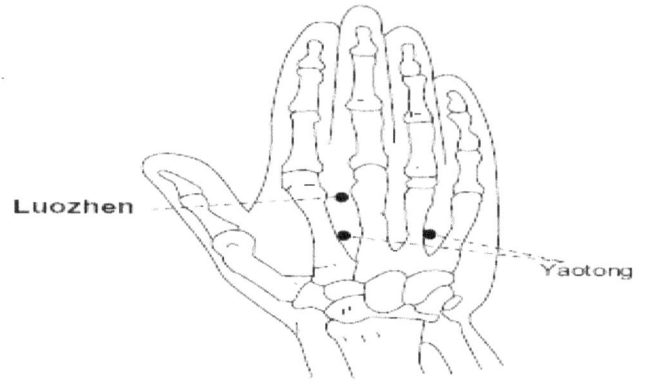

Formula One: Luozhen–Xuanzhong (GB39)

Luozhen: An extra point located at the ulnar side of the second base joint on the dorsum of the hand.

Acupuncture is performed. Insert a needle into the Luozhen point at 0.5–0.8 *cun* deep. Then, insert another needle into the Xuanzhong (GB39) on the affected side at approximately 1.5 *cun* deep. At the same time, ask the patient to move his or her head. After approximately 10 min, the symptoms will be relieved. Remove the needles after 25–30 min. Then, perform cupping therapy.

The practitioner used the Luozhen–Xuanzhong (GB39) points to treat stiff neck in 22 cases. After three sessions of treatment, the efficacy rate was 100%.

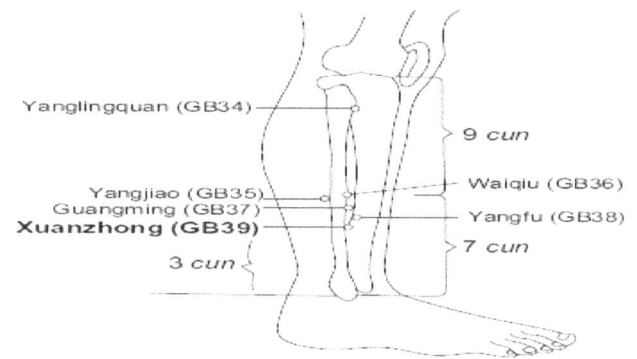

Formula Two: Wanshuner (T 22.09)–Neiguan (PC6)

Wanshuner (T 22.09): An extra point located 5 *fen* beneath the Houxi (SI3). Most practitioners, particularly those who specialize in acupuncture, are more likely to refine their skills and look for more effective acupoints. Seldom, are experts willing to share their experiences. TCM practitioners in Taiwan have special skills in using herbal medicine. However, these practitioners are not like practitioners in mainland China, who are more willing to share their experiences to promote the development of TCM. We are willing to share his experience with other colleagues to promote the development of Chinese acupuncture in Taiwan.

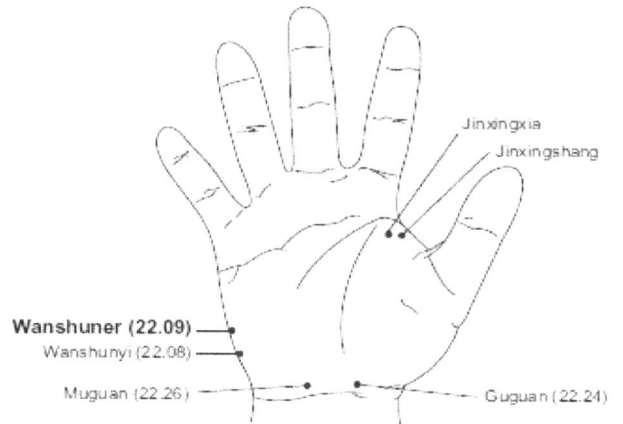

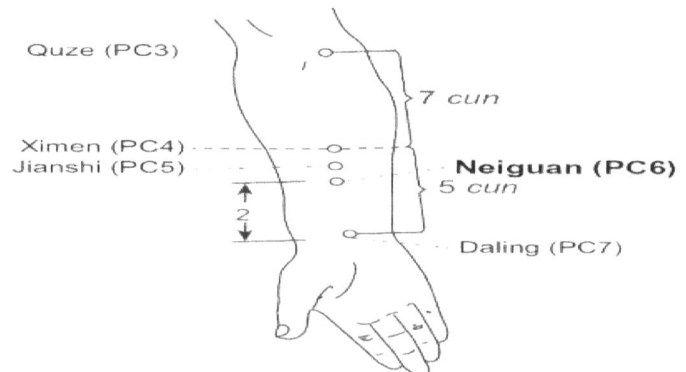

Sprain in the Soft Tissue of the Neck

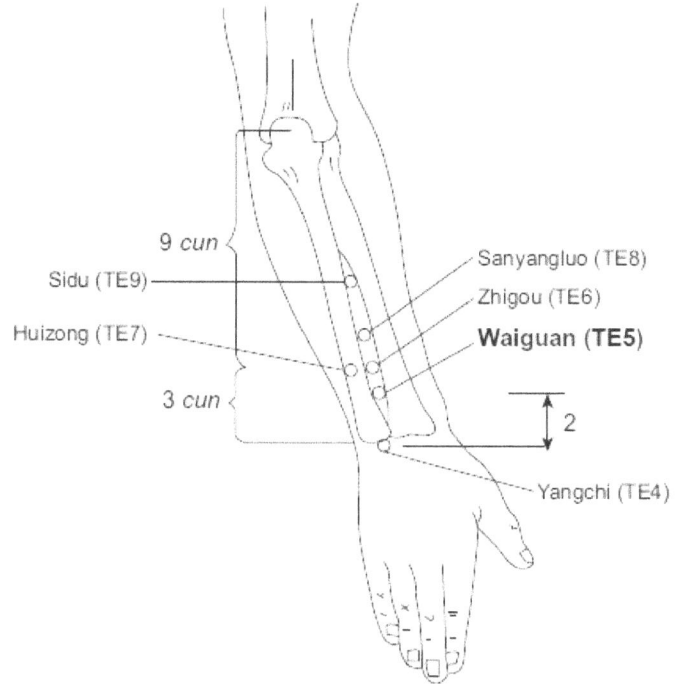

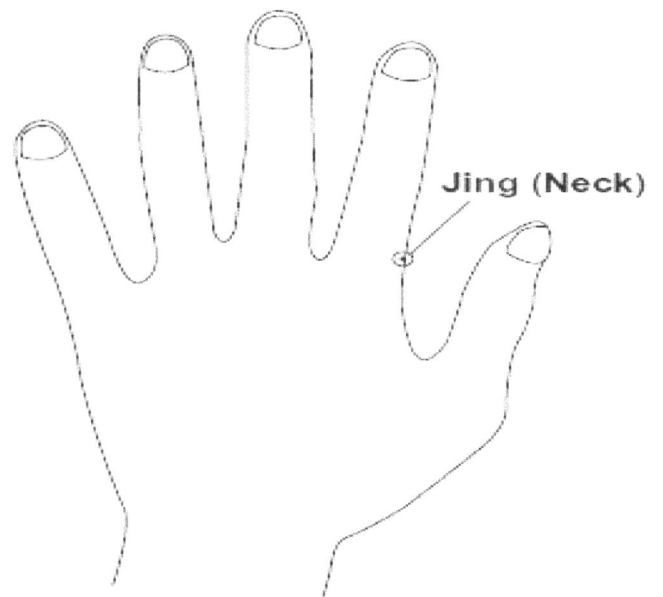

Waiguan (TE5)–Jingdian (hand point)

Jingdian (hand point): Located at the radial side of the second base joint.

Acupuncture is performed. Insert needles perpendicularly without twisting.

Case: Mr. Wang, a 34-year-old man developed a sprain in the neck when driving. The pain lasted for 2 days. Moreover, he had problems with moving his head. After one session of treatment with this method, the symptoms completely disappeared.

Sprain in the Soft Tissue of the Neck

Acute Sprain in the Lower Back

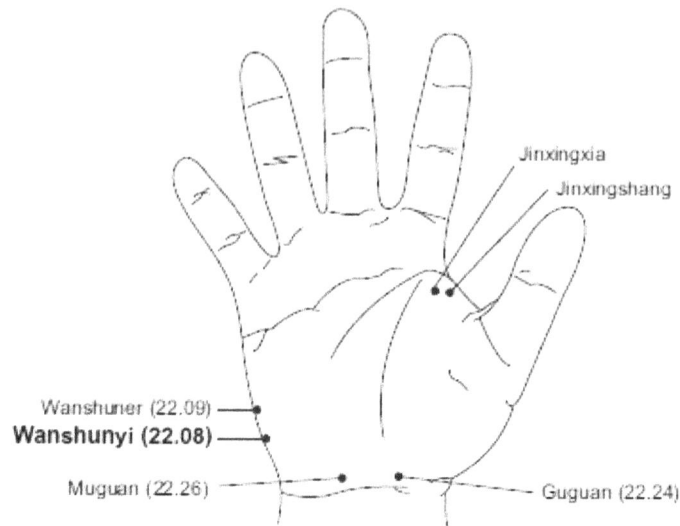

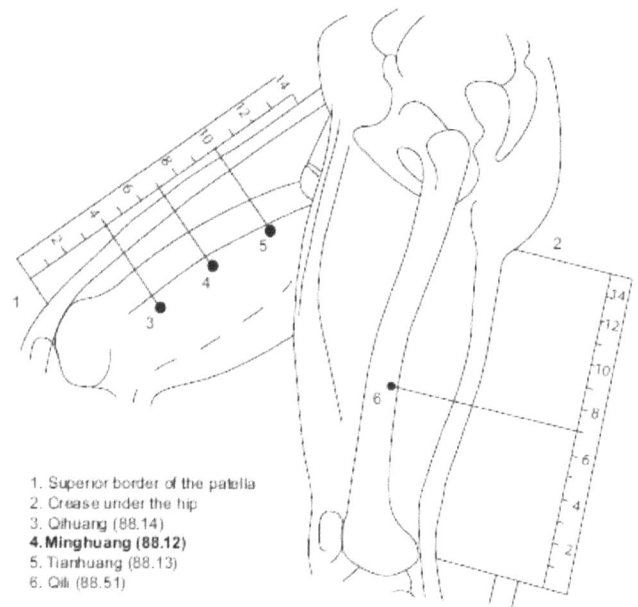

Acute Sprain in the Lower Back

Wanshunyi (T 22.08)–Minghuang (T 88.12)

Acupuncture is performed. Select points on the affected side. Insert needles at 1.5–2 *cun* deep, without any specific needle technique.

The Wanshunyi (T 22.08)–Minghuang (T 88.12) points can be used for treating not only problems in the lumbar vertebrae but also syndromes, such as kidney deficiency and liver fire hyperactivity. If used properly, this pair of points can be effective in relieving pain.

Jinxingxia

Jinxingshang

Wanshuner (22.09)

Wanshunyi (22.08)

Muguan (22.26)

Guguan (22.24)

1. Superior border of the patella
2. Crease under the hip
3. Qihuang (88.14)
4. **Minghuang (88.12)**
5. Tianhuang (88.13)
6. Qili (88.51)

Chest Injury

Neiguan (PC6)–Taixi (KI3)

Acupuncture is performed. Select the Neiguan (PC6)–Taixi (KI3) points were selected. After using the reducing technique and obtaining needle insertion sensation, leave the needles in place for 20–30 min.

We used this method to treat chest pain caused by injury or overwork. Usually, patients come to our clinic after a massage or after taking herbal medicines that are not effective in relieving pain. They present with chest pain when breathing. This pain is accompanied with cough. Patients cannot lie flat on their backs. After one session of treatment, this pain will be relieved. Then, combine this treatment with herbal medicine. The pain will disappear after three sessions of treatment.

Chest Injury

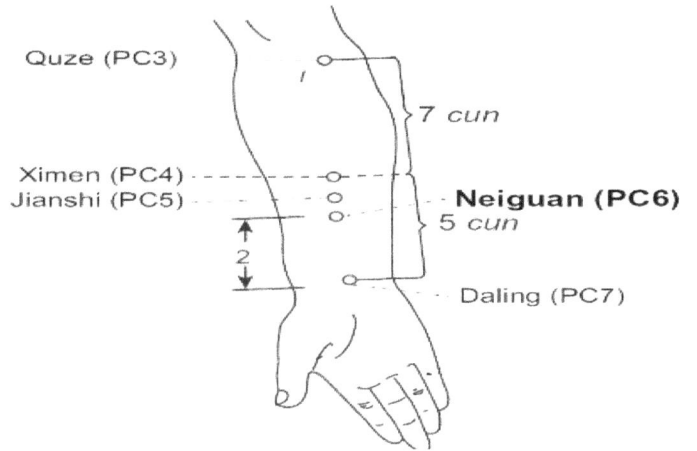

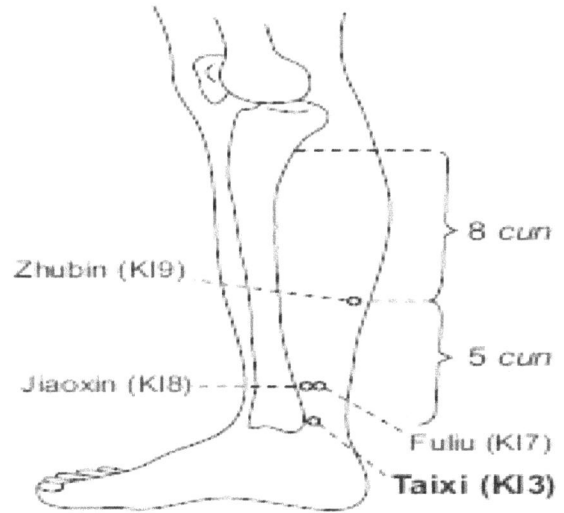

Soft Tissue Injury in the Lower Back and Legs

Dazhui (GV14)–Wangu (SI4)

Acupuncture is performed. Ask the patient to keep standing and to raise his or her arm in front of the body parallel to the floor. Use 0.38-mm needles. Insert a needle upward obliquely into the Dazhui (GV14) at approximately 1 *cun* deep. After obtaining needle insertion sensation, insert needles perpendicularly into the Wangu (SI4) in both hands at approximately 0.5 *cun* deep. Then, manipulate the needles, mainly performing the reducing technique with strong stimulation. Keep manipulating the needle in the Dazhui (GV14) first until the patient feels a sense of electricity radiating to the lower back. Then, manipulate the needles in the Wangu (SI4). The patient can feel pain, tingling, or distension in the points. At the same time, perform the Dong-Qi technique. The intensity of manipulation should be tolerated by the patient. Keep manipulating needles until the patients can squat and stand. Then ask the patient to sit down and leave the needles in place for 30 min. Before removing the needles, manipulate the needles again, as described above.

This method was used to treat soft tissue injury in the lower back and legs in 18 cases. In total, 12 patients were completely treated and improvement was noted in four. However, the method was ineffective in two cases. The efficacy rate was 88.89%.

The Dazhui (GV14) is located in the governing vessel, which passes through the lower back. The utilization of the Wangu (SI4) relieves muscle rigidity and activates the collaterals. It can be used to treat shoulder, arm, and neck pain. Thus, selecting the Dazhui (GV14)–Wangu (SI4) points and using in this treatment method, as described above can treat soft tissue injury in the lower back and legs.

Soft Tissue Injury in the Lower Back and Legs

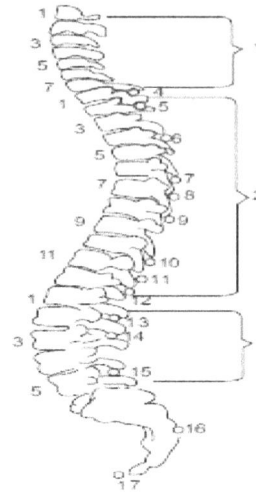

1. Cervical vertebrae
2. Thoracic vertebrae
3. Lumbar vertebrae
4. **Dazhui (GV14)**
5. Taodao (GV13)
6. Shenzhu (GV12)
7. Shendao (GV11)
8. Lingtai (GV10)
9. Zhiyang (GV9)
10. Jinsuo (GV8)
11. Zhongshu (GV7)
12. Jizhong (GV6)
13. Xuanshu (GV5)
14. Mingmen (GV4)
15. Yaoyangguan (GV3)
16. Yaoshu (GV2)
17. Changqiang (GV1)

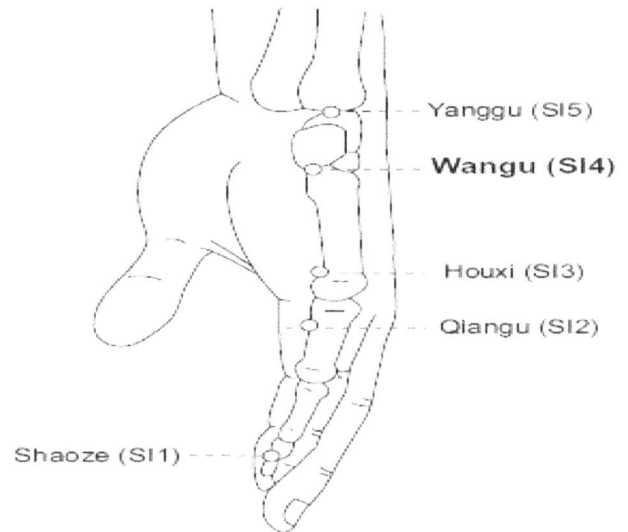

Yanggu (SI5)
Wangu (SI4)
Houxi (SI3)
Qiangu (SI2)
Shaoze (SI1)

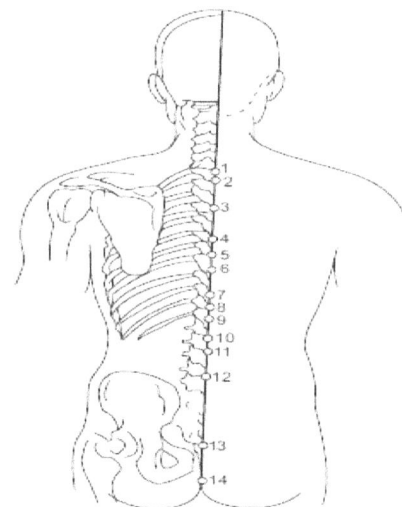

1. Dazhui (GV14)
2. Taodao (GV13)
3. Shenzhu (GV12)
4. Shendao (GV11)
5. Lingtai (GV10)
6. Zhiyang (GV9)
7. Jinsuo (GV8)
8. Zhongshu (GV7)
9. Jizhong (GV6)
10. Xuanshu (GV5)
11. Mingmen (GV4)
12. Yaoyangguan (GV3)
13. Yaoshu (GV2)
14. Changqiang (GV1)

Injury in the Superior Cluneal Nerves

L2 Jiaji (Hua Tuo Jia Ji)–Ashi point

L2 Jiaji: Two extra points located 0.5 *cun* lateral to the L2 spinous process.

Ashi point: Located 2-finger-breadths (1.5 *cun*) beneath the midpoint of the iliac spine.

Acupuncture is performed. Ask the patient to lie on his or her stomach. Select points on the affected side. Use 0.38 × 75-mm needles. Perform the reducing technique. After obtaining the needle insertion sensation, keep manipulating needles until the needle sensation radiates to the affected leg.

In this condition, the affected area is located 2-finger-breadth (1.5 *cun*) beneath the midpoint of the iliac spine, where a string-like node can be felt. The node is painful when pressed. The pain can radiate to the knees and popliteal areas. The acupoint is selected based on "the painful point." This method is effective in relieving pain. However, when this method is combined with electro-acupuncture, its efficacy increases.

Injury in the Superior Cluneal Nerves

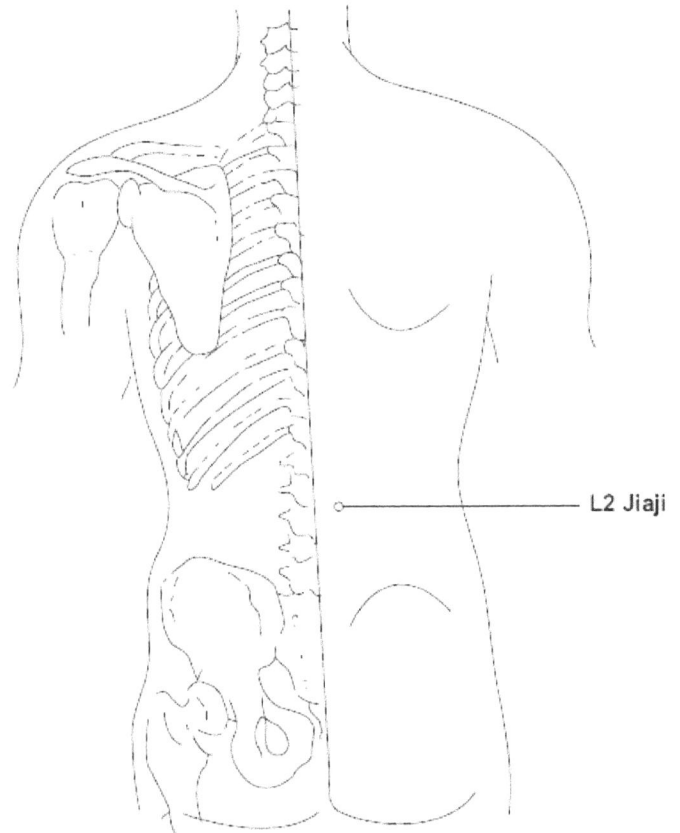

L2 Jiaji

Lumbar Muscle Strain

This condition is often caused by injury or overwork of the lumbar muscle. Moreover, it can be caused by exogenous phenomena that could block channels and obstruct the circulation of Qi and blood. Thus, this condition is often accompanied with strain in the teres major. The tender point is near the Tianzong (SI11).

Formula One: Tianzong (SI11)–Shenguan (T 77.18)

Acupuncture is performed to treat strain in the teres major. The treatment can be immediately effective in relieving pain.

Case: Ms. Shanqi, a 40-year-old woman, suffered from arm pain for 5 years. The pain was progressive. The patient had problems with flexion and extension, and she could not raise her arms. The muscles on the affected side were atrophic. Treatments with massage and block therapy were ineffective.

After two sessions of treatment with this method, the pain disappeared, and her bodily functions were restored.

Formula Two: Weiling–Taichong (LR3)

Weiling: An extra point located 1.5 *cun* beneath the wrist crease, between the 2nd and the 3rd metacarpal bones, and at the radial side of the 2nd tendon of the extensor digitorum.

This method is extremely effective in relieving pain and is highly recommended when used to treat problems in the lumbar area.

Lumbar Muscle Strain

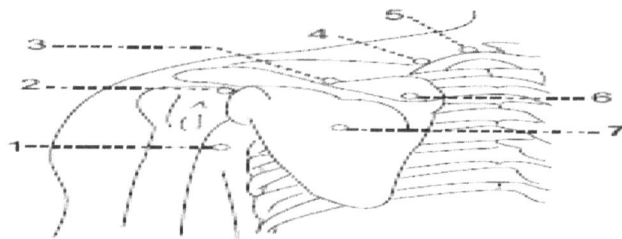

1. Jianzhen (SI9)
2. Naoshu (SI10)
3. Bingfeng (SI12)
4. Jianwaishu (SI14)
5. Jianzhongshu (SI15)
6. Quyuan (SI13)
7. Tianzong (SI11)

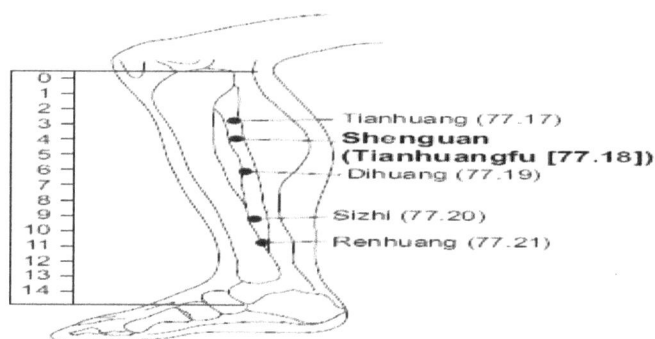

Tianhuang (77.17)
Shenguan (Tianhuangfu [77.18])
Dihuang (77.19)
Sizhi (77.20)
Renhuang (77.21)

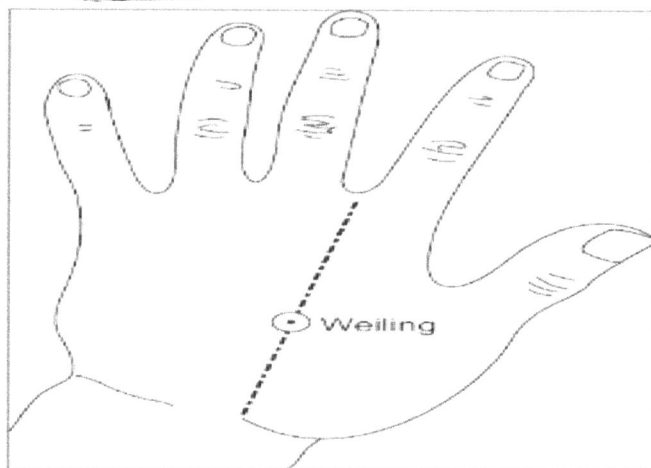

Weiling

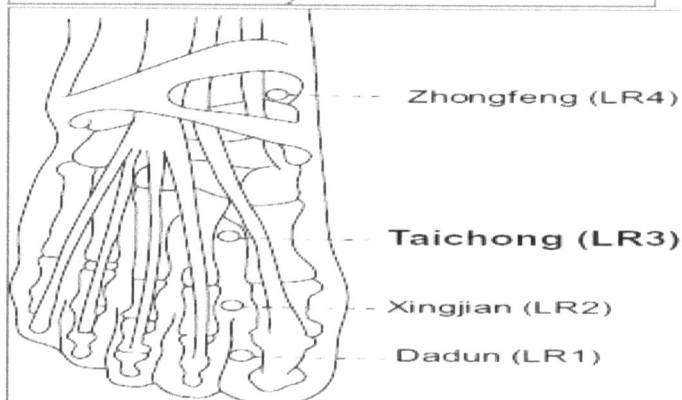

Zhongfeng (LR4)

Taichong (LR3)

Xingjian (LR2)

Dadun (LR1)

Sprain in the Joints

Mingmen (GV4)–Qiuxu (GB40)

The Mingmen (GV4)–Qiuxu (GB40) points were used for treating sprain in the joints in 100 cases. In total, 97 cases were cured, where the pain and swelling disappeared, active function was restored, and the patients were able to work or exercise after treatment. Two cases improved (reduced swelling and pain). However, the treatment method was ineffective in one case. The total efficacy rate was 97%.

Case: Sandra, a 34-year-old Mexican woman, sprained her lower back twice during work. On examination tenderness beside the L4 and L5 vertebrae was observed when bending down. After one session of treatment, pain and limitation of movement disappeared.

Acupoints are selected according to affected areas and channels using this method. It is significantly effective in treating sprain. After air enters the acupoints, the stimulation spreads through the channels. It can activate the Qi and blood, dissipate blood stasis, and reduce swelling.

Sprain in the Joints

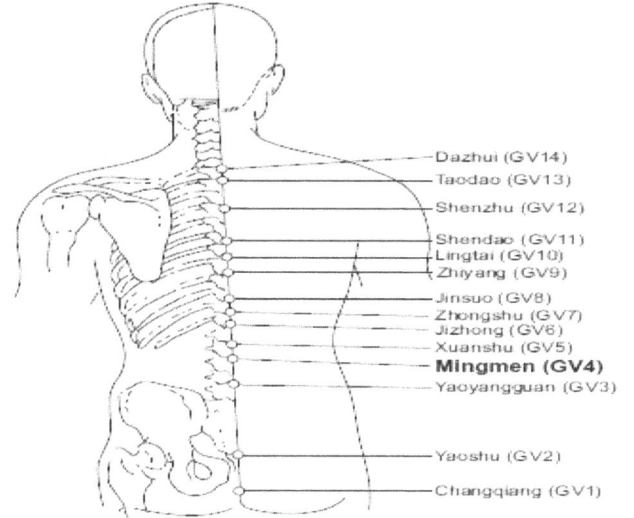

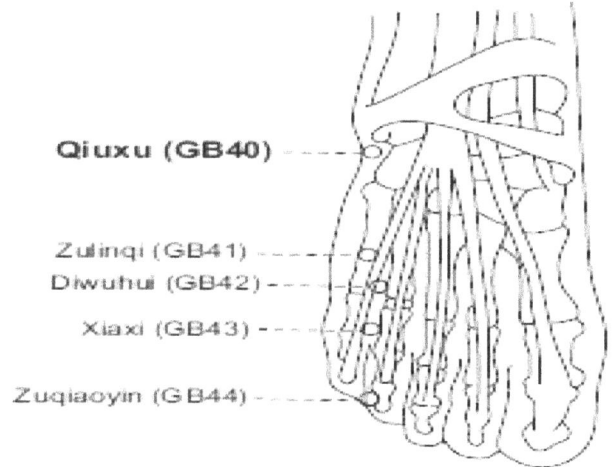

Sprain in the Wrist
Taixi (KI3)–Shangjiaoqu (lip point)

Acupuncture is performed. Leave needles in place for 20–30 min.

The Taixi (KI3)–Shangjiaoqu points are used for treating sprains in the wrist. It can alleviate pain within a short period of time. However, syndrome differentiation and diagnosis should be confirmed before using this pair of points.

In the theory of Dong's extra points, the corresponding points in the hands and feet can also be used, which is called the Yin–Yang balance needling technique. As long as the right points are selected, the treatment can be effective in treating the sprain.

Sprain in the Wrist

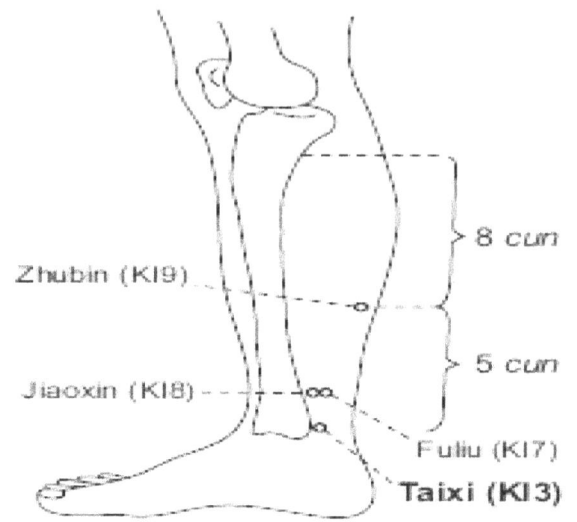

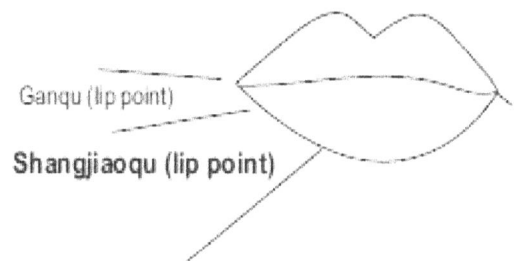

The location of lip point is on the adjunct of red lip and skin

34

Sprain in the Ankle

Xiayiqu–Xiaerqu (wrist–ankle extra points)

Xiayiqu and Xiaerqu are the extra points in the wrist and ankle, respectively. If you are interested in this field, there are other books that can be used as reference.

Acupuncture is performed. Use 0.32 × 40 mm or 0.28 × 40 mm needles. Insert needles obliquely, enabling the needles and skin to form a 30° angle. Leave needles in place for 30 min without twisting.

Case: Michael Zhang, a 23-year old man, sprained his ankle when playing a ball game. His ankle was red, swollen, and painful. He could not walk. Moreover, he used a pain-relieving patch. However, treatment was ineffective. He was treated with this method four times. Then, he could move his ankle again. After taking two doses of herbal medicine, he was completely cured.

Sprain in the Ankle

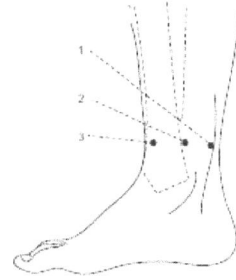

1. Xia1: on the medial border of tendo calcaneus, 3 finger length above the top of medial malleolus
2. Xia2: on the middle of the inner side of leg, posterior border of tibia, 3 finger length above the top of medial malleolus
3. Xia3: 1 cm in front of the anterior border of tibia, 3 finger length above the top of medial malleolus

Knee Arthritis due to Sprain

Yanglingquan (GB34)–Shaohai (HT3)

Acupuncture is performed with moderate stimulation. Leave needles in place for 20 min and manipulating the needles once every 10 min.

This method was used for treating knee arthritis due to injury in three cases. It was effective in treating the sprain after one session of treatment in all cases.

Knee Arthritis due to Sprain

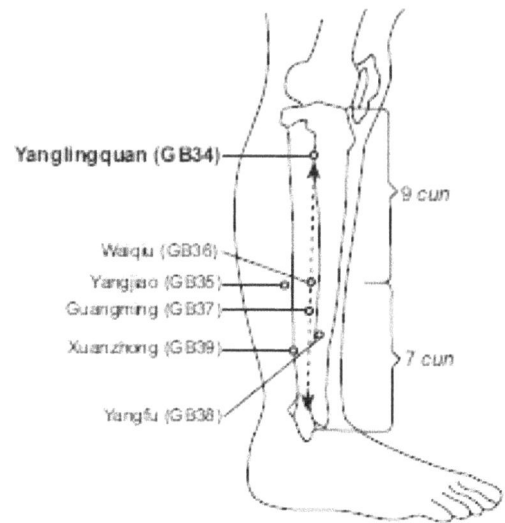

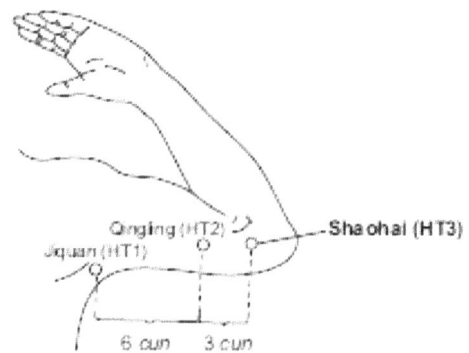

Chapter Three

Orthopedic Diseases and Traumatology

Cervical Spondylosis

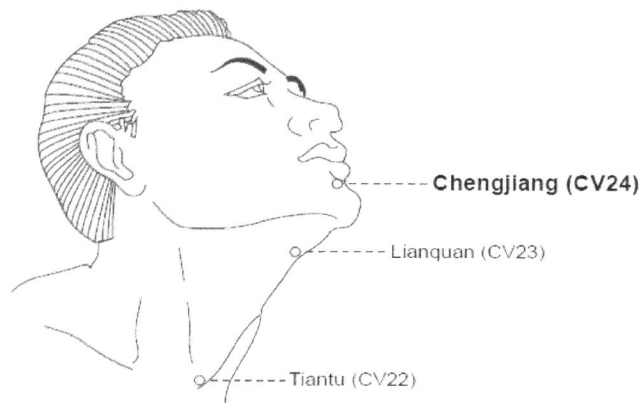

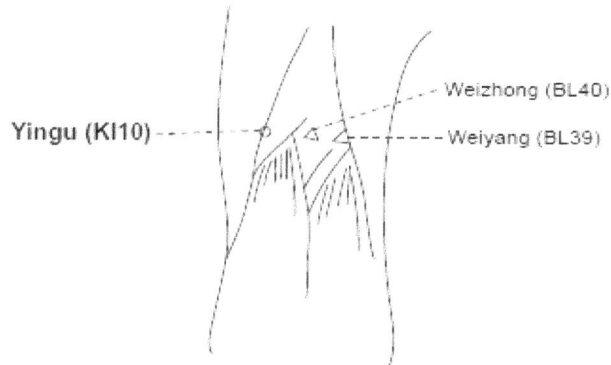

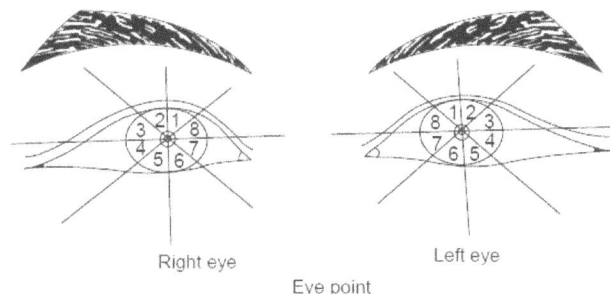

Cervical spondylosis is often caused by poor sleeping position, common cold, bad weather, injury, and degeneration.

There are many reasons for neck pain, including a stiff neck, acute soft tissue injury, and myofascial syndrome. Practitioners should determine the pair of points after confirming the diagnosis.

Formula One: Chengjiang (CV24)–Yingu (KI10)

Acupuncture is performed. Insert the needles perpendicularly, performing a controlled needle technique. This method can improve motion limitation caused by cervical spondylosis.

Formula Two: Shangjiaoqu (Eye point)–Xiaochangqu (Eye point)

Acupuncture with filiform needles is performed. After achieving needle insertion sensation, leave the needles in place for 15 min, manipulating the needles once every 5 min. This method is very effective for reliving neck pain caused by cervical spondylosis.

Cervical Spondylosis

Chengjiang (CV24)

Lianquan (CV23)

Tiantu (CV22)

Yingu (KI10)

Weizhong (BL40)

Weiyang (BL39)

Right eye

Left eye

Eye point

1. Fei Dachang (Lung and Large Intestine)
2. Shen Pangguang (Kidney and Bladder)
3. Shangjiao (Upper Energizer)
4. Gandan (Liver and Gallbladder)
5. Zhongjiao (Middle Energizer)
6. Xin Xiaochang (Heart and Small Intestine)
7. Piwei (Spleen and Stomach)
8. Xiajiao (Lower Energizer)

Strain in the Neck Muscle

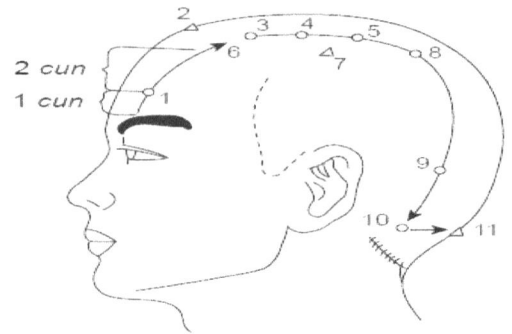

Fengchi (GB20)–Jianjing (GB21)

Acupuncture is performed. Strongly stimulate the Jianjing (GB21). Leave the needle in place for 30 min at the Fengchi (GB20). Simultaneously, perform bloodletting therapy. After one session of treatment, the disease can be cured.

Strain in the Neck Muscle

1. Yangbai (GB14)
2. Shenting (GV24)
3. Toulinqi (GB15)
4. Muchuang (GB16)
5. Zhengying (GB17)
6. Benshen (GB13)
7. Touwei (ST8)
8. Chengling (GB18)
9. Naokong (GB19)
10. **Fengchi (GB20)**
11. Fengfu (GV16)

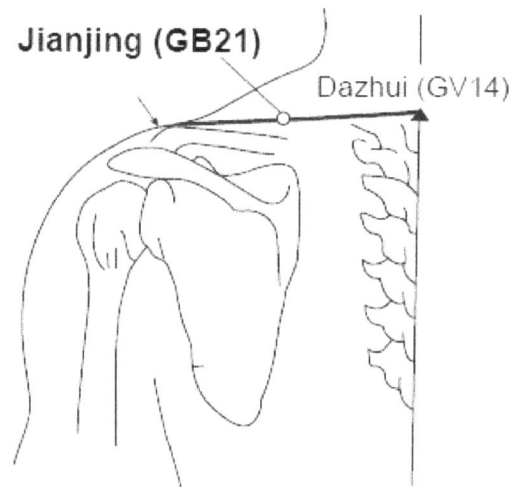

Jianjing (GB21)

Dazhui (GV14)

Cervical Hyperosteogeny

Cervical Hyperosteogeny

Guanyuan (CV4)–Yanglingquan (GB34)

Acupuncture is performed. The Guanyuan (CV4) and Yanglingquan (GB34) are selected. This method is also called the heaven–earth needle technique. Ask the patient to lie on his/her back. Insert the needles perpendicularly at 0.5–1 *cun* deep. After achieving the needle insertion sensation, leave the needles in place for 20 min.

Case: Ms. Wang, a 45-year-old woman, suffered from neck pain with limited motion for 3 weeks. Muscles of her right shoulder often ached. Her left arm tingled and she experienced numbness and weakness, with the sensation spreading to the ring finger and little finger of her left hand. X-ray showed cervical hyperosteogeny. The day after treatment, she could move her head normally and felt 80% relief of shoulder and arm pain. After two more sessions of treatments, all symptoms disappeared.

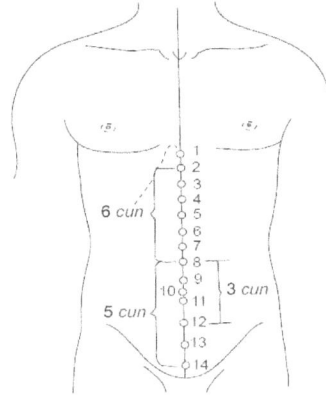

1. Jiuwei (CV15)
2. Juque (CV14)
3. Shangwan (CV13)
4. Zhongwan (CV12)
5. Jianli (CV11)
6. Xiawan (CV10)
7. Shuifen (CV9)
8. Shenque (CV8)
9. Yinjiao (CV7)
10. Qihai (CV6)
11. Shimen (CV5)
12. **Guanyuan (CV4)**
13. Zhongji (CV3)
14. Qugu (CV2)

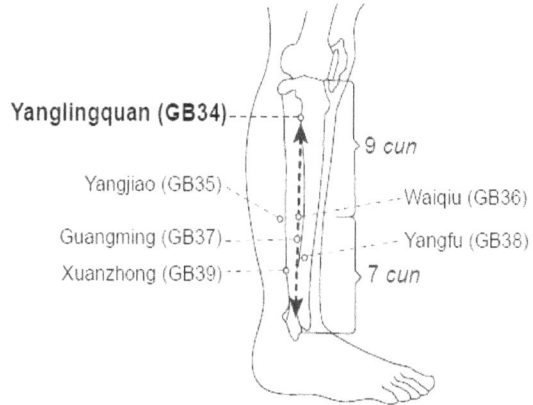

Scalenus Anticus Syndrome

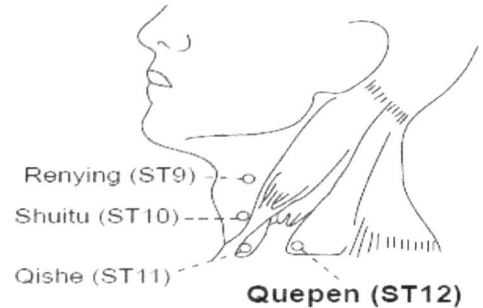

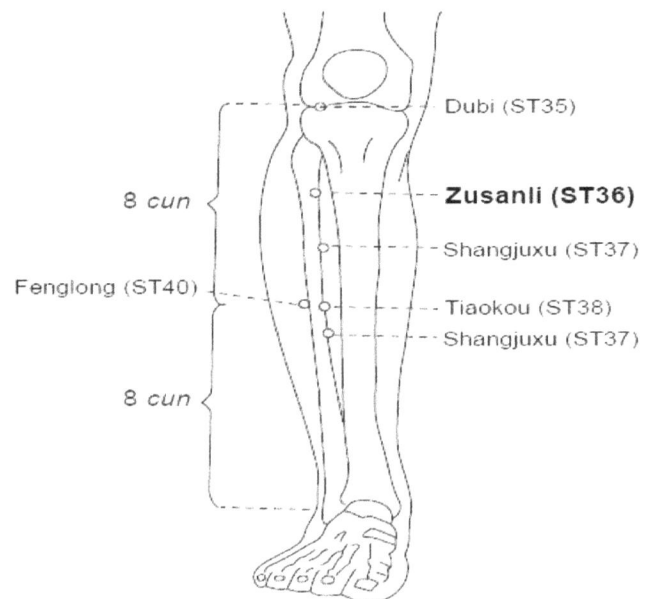

Quepen (ST12)–Zusanli (ST36)

Acupuncture is performed. Insert the needles perpendicularly at 1.5 *cun* deep. Leave the needles in place for 30 min. Perform treatment once a day for 10 days. Usually, the patient will feel improvement after one session of treatment.

Mr. Zhang, a 24-year-old man, developed pain in the scalenus anticus after lifting a weight. The pain radiated to the inside of the upper arm and ulnar side of the forearm and hand. It was accompanied by tingling, numbness, and distension. The occiput area was sometimes affected and he could not sleep. Examination showed tenderness in the supraclavicular fossa and muscle tension. Right scalenus anticus syndrome was diagnosed in the patient. After 10 sessions with this method, he was cured. During treatment, a triangular bandage was used to hang the affected arm. He was recommended to dress in warm clothes and cover his neck.

Scalenus Anticus Syndrome

Renying (ST9)
Shuitu (ST10)
Qishe (ST11)
Quepen (ST12)

Dubi (ST35)
8 *cun*
Zusanli (ST36)
Shangjuxu (ST37)
Fenglong (ST40)
Tiaokou (ST38)
Shangjuxu (ST37)
8 *cun*

Periarthritis of the Shoulder

Periarthritis of the Shoulder

Acupuncture for periarthritis of the shoulder is recorded in many ancient books. It was first recorded by Huangfu Mi in the Jin Dynasty (266–420 A.D.) in his book Zhenjiu Jiayi jing. He said that shoulder pain with problem in raising the arm can be treated with the Tianrong (SI17) and Bingfeng (SI12) points. In modern times, practitioners use many acupoints to treat this disease, including Dong's extra points such as the Fanhoujue (22.12) and Shenguan (77.18). Treatment at these points is immediately effective. Here are other pairs of points for your reference.

Formula One: Quepen (ST12)–Yexia

Yexia: An extra point located at the midpoint of the latissimus dorsi. Acupuncture is performed. Insert a needle into the Quepen (ST12) at a depth of 0.5–1 *cun*. The needle insertion sensation will spread to the thumb and index finger. Insert another needle into the Yexia, with the needle pointing to the acromion. Insert this needle at a depth of 2–2.5 *cun*. Simultaneously, ask the patient to raise his/her arm. Perform the Dong Qi needle technique and lift the needle beneath the skin. Ask the patient to lower his/her arm, and then raise his/her arm again. Then, insert the needle and manipulate it. Repeat this process three times. Perform this treatment once daily for 10 days. Normally, the disease will be cured after 10 days.

Formula Two: Tiaokou (ST38)–Lingxia

Lingxia: An extra point located 2 *cun* under the Yanglingquan (GB34). Acupuncture is performed with a needle measuring 0.38 × 100 mm. Insert the needle deeply into the Tiaokou (ST38) on the unaffected side, with the needle penetrating the Chengshan (BL57). Perform the Dong-Qi needle technique. Normally, after achieving the needle insertion sensation, it is immediately effective.

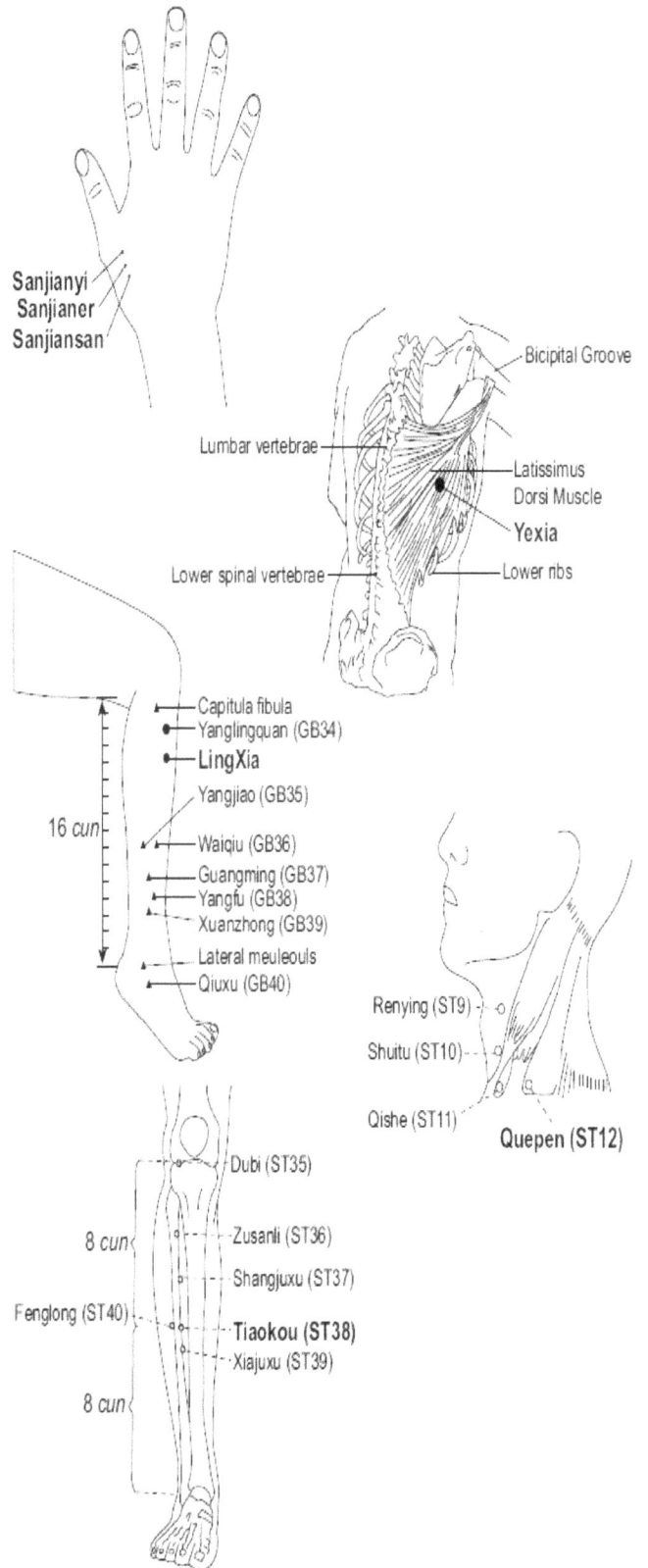

Lateral Epicondylitis

Formula One: Ashi point–Taixi (KI3)

Acupuncture is performed. Insert the needles into the
Taixi (KI3). Prepare herbal medicine as follows:
Shexiang (musk), 1 g; Zhangnao (camphor), 10 g; Xuejie
(draconis resin), 3 g; Ercha (cutch), 3 g; Chuanwu
(common monkshood mother root), 3 g; and Caowu
(Kusnezoff monkshood root), 3 g. Mix these herbs and
crush them into a powder. Store the powder in a small
bottle for future usage. Mix flour and water to make
dough. Then, roll the dough to form a noodle. Put the
noodle on the tenderness point of the lateral epicondyle of
the humerus to make a 1.5-cm–diameter circle. Then,
apply a layer (as thick as a coin) of the prepared herbal
medicine powder into the circle. Cut a moxa stick into
shorter 1.5-cm-long sticks. Put one stick on the herbal
powder and ignite it. Moxibustion should not cause
burning. For the Taixi (KI3), use three moxa cones for
moxibustion. Most patients will be cured after one session
of treatment. This method is miraculous. We share it here
for reference.

Lateral Epicondylitis

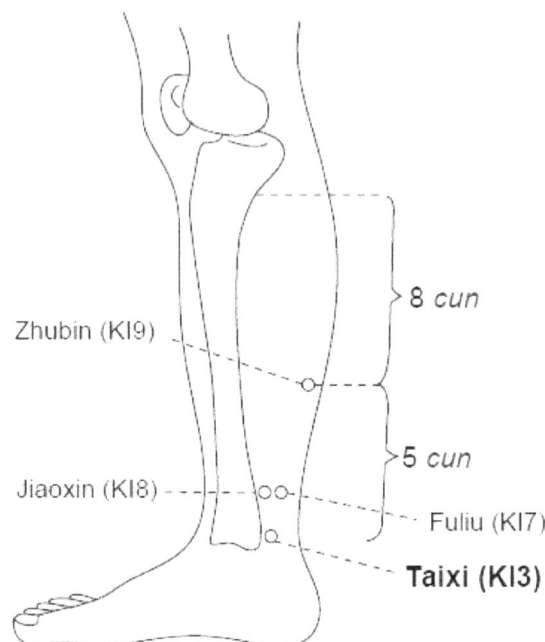

Zhubin (KI9)

8 cun

5 cun

Jiaoxin (KI8)

Fuliu (KI7)

Taixi (KI3)

42

Thecal Cyst

Thecal Cyst

Kongzui (LU6)–Waiguan (TE5)

Acupuncture is performed on the Kongzui (LU6) and Waiguan (TE5). Triple needling is performed. Place a medicine cake made of Fuzi (common monkshood branched root) on the points. Use moxa cones to perform moxibustion. When the skin turns red, stop moxibustion. This therapy should not cause blisters or burns.

This method was used to treat a thecal cyst in one case. After three sessions of treatments, the pain stopped completely and the cyst disappeared.

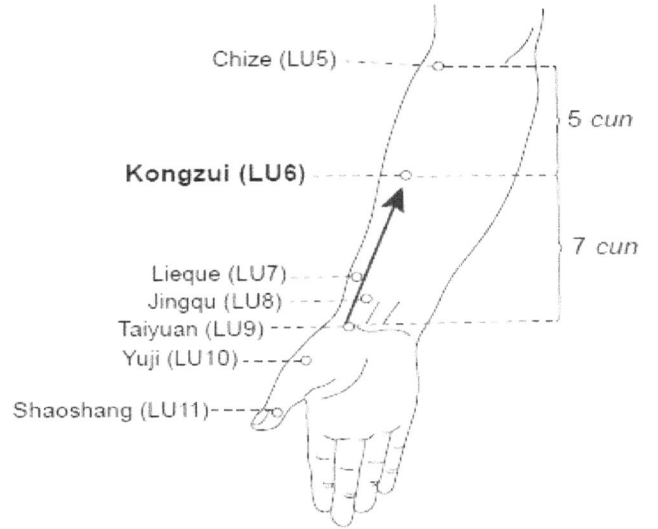

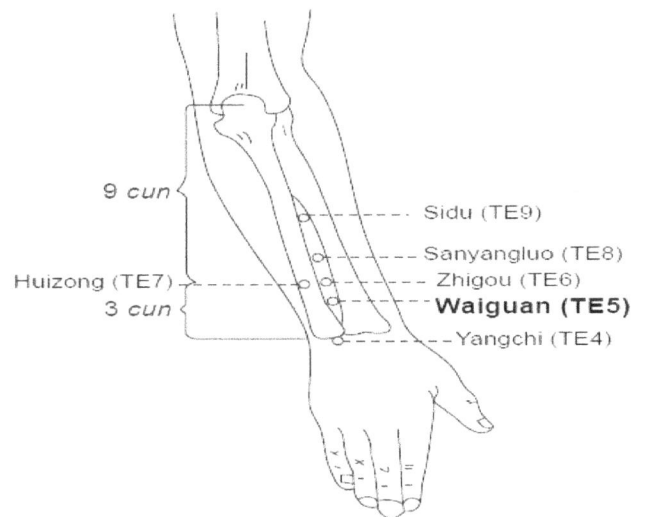

Tenosynovitis

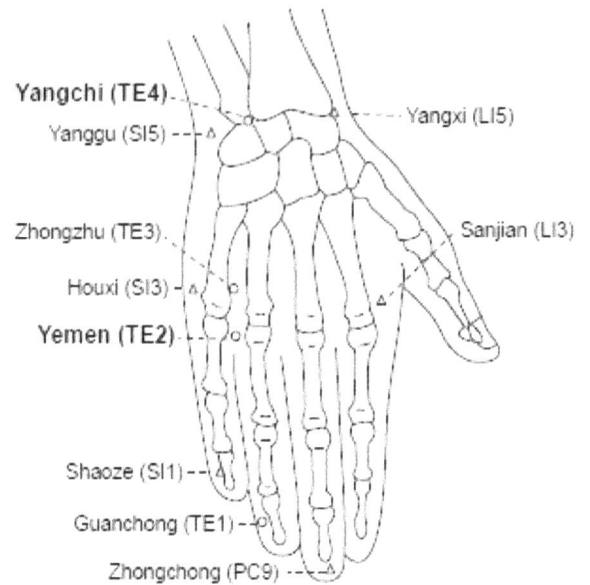

Tenosynovitis

Yemen (TE2)–Yangchi (TE4)

Acupuncture is performed. Insert the needles into the Yemen (TE2) and Yangchi (TE4), performing the uniform reinforcing–reducing technique. Leave the needles in place for 20 min.

The Yangchi (TE4) is located at the transverse crease of the dorsum of the wrist in a depression on the ulnar side of the extensor digitorum communis tendon. It is on the Triple energizer channel, which is a hand Shaoyang channel. In mainland China, acupoint injection is usually performed on this point. With acupoint injection, the patient can benefit from not only the effect of the acupoint but also the effect of the medicine.

During treatment, movement of the affected area should be limited. It is important to keep the area warm and protect it from cold and dampness.

Osteomyelitis

Osteomyelitis

Waiguan (TE5)–Baxie (EX-UE9)

Baxie (EX-UE9): A set of eight extra points on the dorsum of both hands, proximal to the margin of the webs between the fingers.

Moxibustion combined with acupuncture is performed. Wash the wound with normal saline. Insert the needles into the Waiguan (TE5) and Baxie (EX-UE9). After manipulating and achieving the needle insertion sensation, leave the needles in place for 15 min. It is better to have the needle insertion sensation radiating to the fingertips. After removing the needles, put 20 g of moxa wool into a moxibustion box and ignite it. Fumigate the affected area for 30 min and then bind up the wound. Perform the treatment once a day for 7 days. Most patients' symptoms will improve in 7 days.

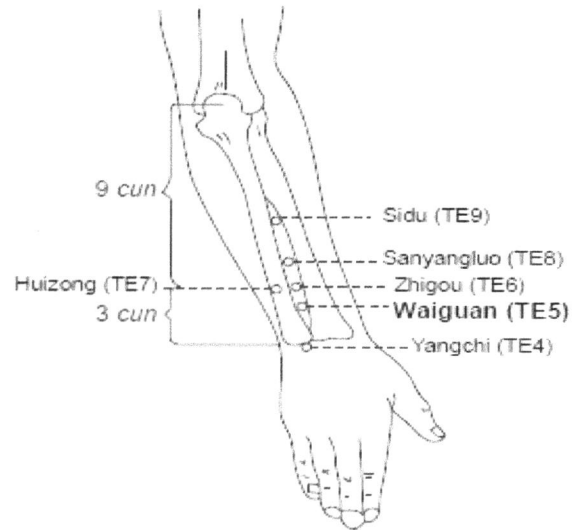

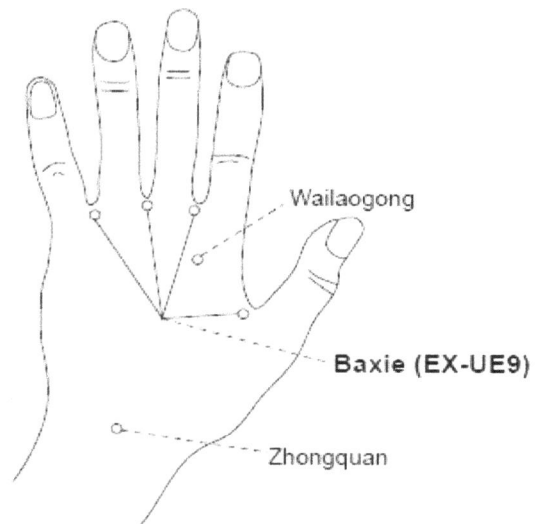

Costochondritis

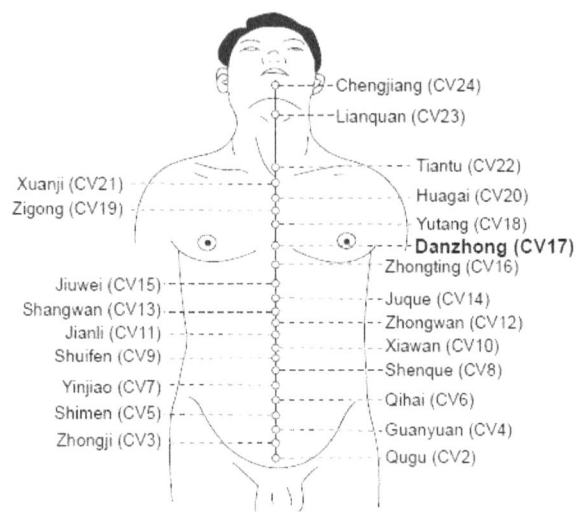

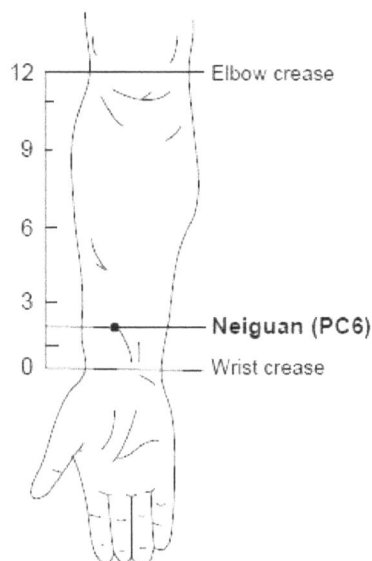

Costochondritis

Danzhong (CV17)–Neiguan (PC6)

Acupuncture is performed. Insert the needles into the points on the affected side, performing the reducing technique with moderate stimulation. Leave the needles in place for 20 min. Twist and twirl the needles once every 1–2 min to maintain the needle insertion sensation. Perform this treatment every other day.

Case: Mr. Chen, a 55-year-old man, developed chest pain 2 years ago. The pain developed between the third and fourth ribs near the sternum. Sometimes it was a dull pain, but sometimes it was a stabbing pain. The pain was recurrent and worsened over 2 years. He took western and Chinese patent medicine and underwent acupuncture many times. However, his pain did not improve. He visited our clinic based on recommendations from his friends. We diagnosed him with costochondritis and treated him with this method. After two sessions of treatments, his pain was relieved. After seven sessions of treatments, the pain disappeared. To consolidate the effect, we performed one more session of treatment. This is presented here for reference.

Thoracic Facet Joint Disturbance Syndrome

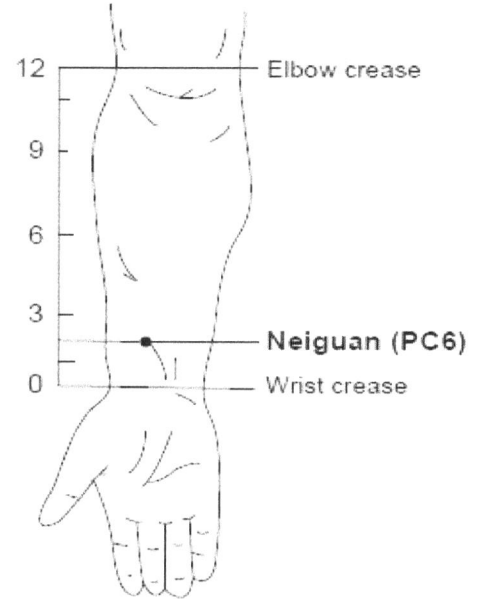

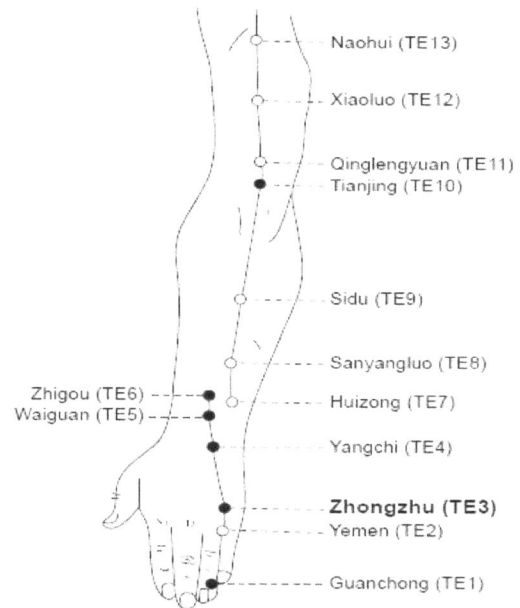

Thoracic Facet Joint Disturbance Syndrome

Thoracic facet joint disturbance syndrome can cause back pain with a sensation of heaviness and discomfort. The pain may be accompanied by pressure in the chest, which can affect deep breathing. It can cause headaches and limit head movement. Tenderness points are also present on and near the thoracic spinous process.

Neiguan (PC6)–Zhongzhu (TE3)

Acupuncture is performed. Insert 50-mm needles and perform strong stimulation. Do not leave the needles in place. Massage can be performed before acupuncture. Ask the patient to lie on his/her stomach. Find the tender point on the back. Put the right hand on the tenderness point and the left hand on the right one. Press the point 3–5 times. Subsequently, perform acupuncture.

Lumbar Disc Herniation

Yinmen (BL37)–Wangu (SI4)

Acupuncture is performed. Select acupoints on the affected side. Insert the needles superficially. After achieving the needle insertion sensation, perform heat-producing needling for 5 min. Perform this therapy once a day. We used this method for treating a case of lumbar disk herniation. The disease was cured after five sessions of treatment.

Case: Wang, a 51-year-old driver, suffered from recurrent left leg pain for 3 years. He took pain relievers and herbal medicines, but the pain did not disappear. The pain worsened after overworking or catching a cold. An X-ray showed tenderness at a point 2 cm left of the L4 and L5 spinous process and at the midpoint of the left hip. The straight leg raising test was positive. He was cured after five sessions of treatment.

This treatment can produce heat in the local area or promote sweating. It is related to stimulation of thermal receptors Krause's corpuscles in the skin. During the treatment, inserting, twisting, and twirling the needle can affect connective tissue and stimulate Krause's corpuscles, producing a warm sensation. For those who are sensitive, the warm sensation may spread through the nerves and cause sweating. In areas rich in soft tissue, the efficacy rate of this method is high. However, for elderly people or those with areas lacking soft tissues, the efficacy rate is low.

Lumbar Disc Herniation

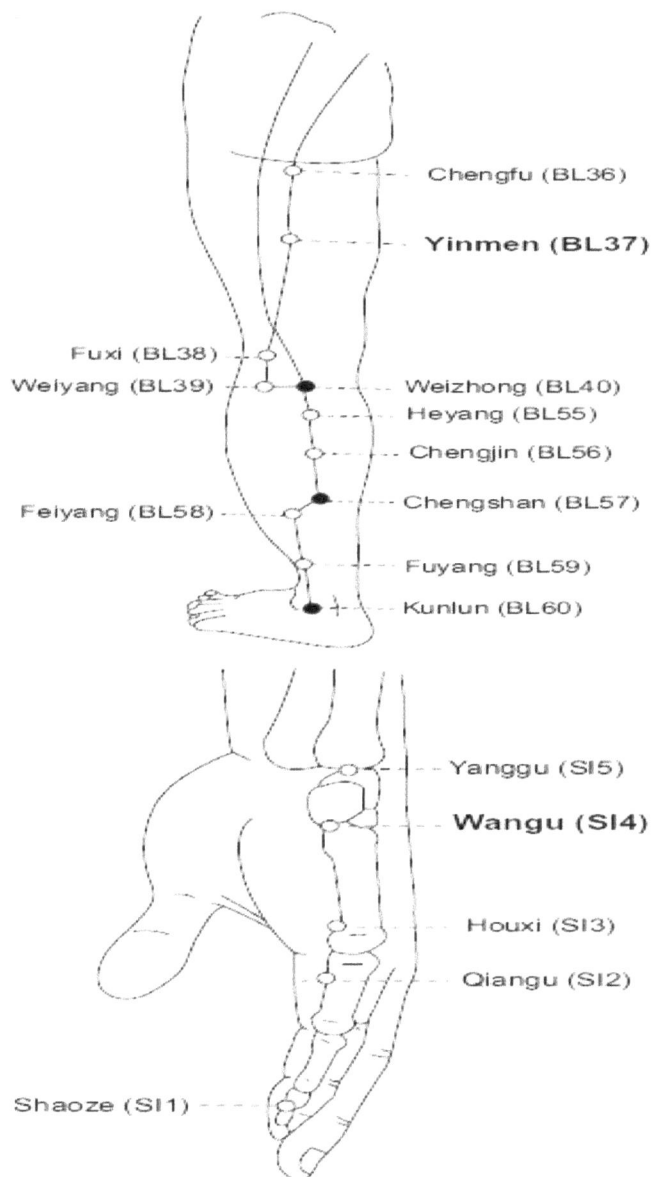

Hyperosteogeny in the Lumbar Vertebrae

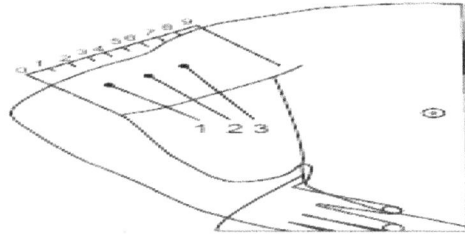

Hyperosteogeny in the Lumbar Vertebrae

Formula One: Guci–Xuehai (SP10)

Guci: An extra point located 4 *cun* above the Quchi (LI11). Ask the patient to hunch his or her back. The Guci is located at the midpoint of the Jianyu (LI15) and Quchi (LI11) acupoints.

Guci is a point identified by Mr. Dong and is one of his secret points. Insert a needle into Guci at 5–8 *fen* deep. Leave the needle in place for 30 min. This method is used for treating hyperosteogeny in the lumbar vertebrae. The disease is common in people aged 40–60 years. Both men and women can develop this disease. The patient cannot straighten his or her lumbar vertebrae because of hyperosteogeny, which is bothersome. Besides acupuncture, wrapping the waist with a magnetic belt to reduce lumbar load can be very helpful.

Formula Two: Erjiaoming (11.12)–Shenguan (77.18)

This pair of points is commonly used by Mr. Dong's students for treating lower back pain. Usually, as long as the right points are selected and used properly, treatment is effective immediately. This pair of points can also be used for treating diseases on the Governor Vessel and Conception Vessel. Treatment and manipulation of this pair of points is seldom shared with the public, except when teaching face to face.

1. Guci (44.24) 1
2. Guci (44.24) 2
3. Guci (44.24) 3

Xuehai (SP10)

Jimen (SP11)

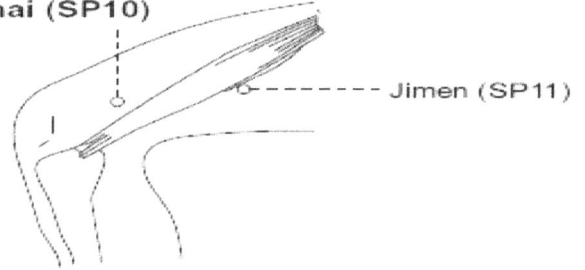

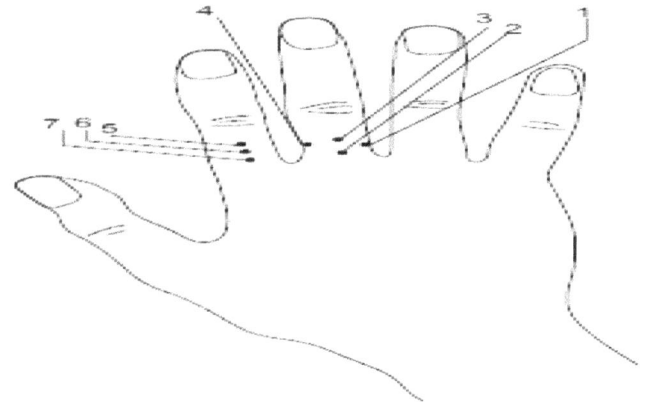

1. Dan (11.13) 2
2. Erjiaoming (11.12) 1
3. Erjiaoming (11.12) 2
4. Dan (11.13) 1
5. Sanxiansan
6. Sanxianer
7. Sanxianyi

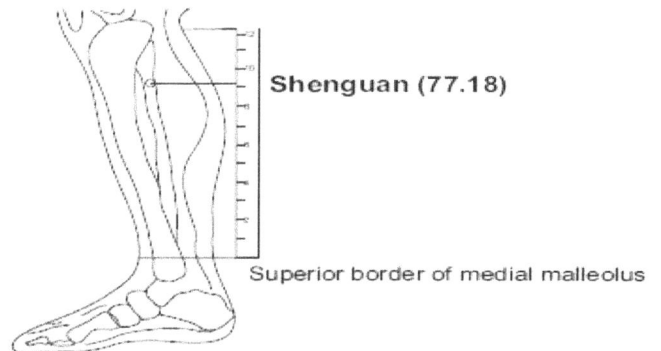

Shenguan (77.18)

Superior border of medial malleolus

The Third Lumbar Transverse Process Syndrome

Weizhong (BL40)–Ashi

Acupuncture is performed. Ask the patient to lie on his or her stomach. Select the Weizhong (BL40) and tenderness point near the third lumbar transverse process. After sterilizing the skin, insert the needles deeply with strong stimulation. After achieving the needle insertion sensation, leave the needles in place for 15–20 min.

Common practitioners seldom use the Ashi points for deep insertion. Some practitioners (Bagua Shenzhen) have reported on inserting the needle 4 *cun* into the lumbar disc and getting a good effect. However, we do not suggest doing so, unless you know the anatomy very well to prevent injury.

We have used this method for treating patients with third lumbar transverse process syndrome. The pain is greatly relieved after one session of treatment. If acupuncture is combined with massage, the pain can completely disappear after three sessions of treatment.

The Third Lumbar Transverse Process Syndrome

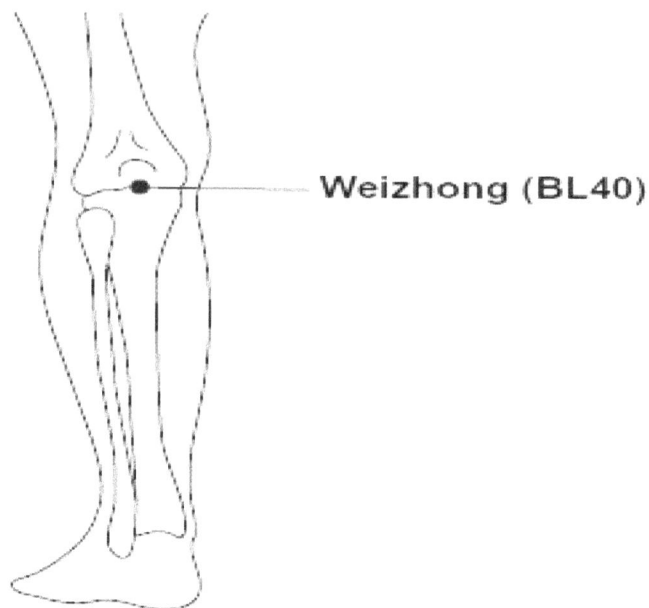

Weizhong (BL40)

Huantiao (GB30)–Zuogu

Zuogu: Located 1 *cun* beneath the midpoint of the greater trochanter and coccyx. Acupuncture is performed. Select the Zuogu as the main point. Insert a needle perpendicularly into the Zuogu, with the needle penetrating to the Zhibian (BL54). Select the Huantiao (GB30) as the supporting point.

Case: Shankou, a 45-year-old woman, developed constricted hip pain 1 month ago after standing up from a squatting position. She used various patches (pain relieving medical plaster with Chinese herbal paste), but no relief could be obtained. She could not lie with her leg straight and found it difficult to walk. Pain radiated to the outer thigh and became worse when coughing. She had obvious tenderness on the right piriformis. Tension test of piriformis was positive. We diagnosed piriformis syndrome in the patient and treated her with this method. After three sessions of treatment, the pain disappeared.

This disease is related to the sacral plexus of the sciatic nerve. Inserting a needle into the Huantiao (GB30) can stimulate the nerve. Inserting a needle into the Zuogu can enhance this effect. This technique is also called Daoma needling.

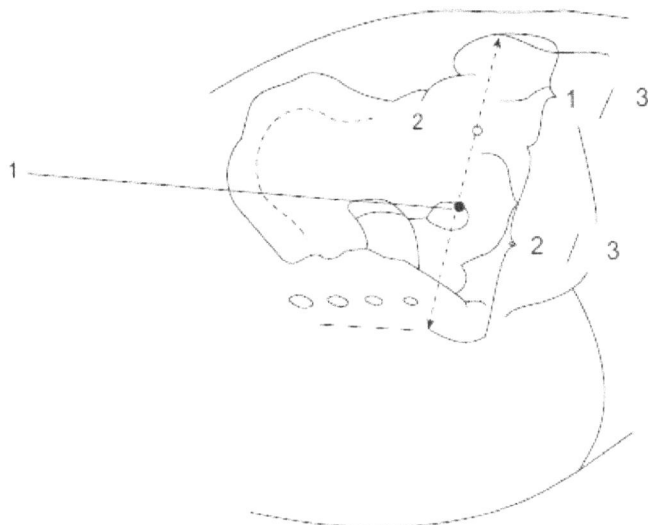

1. Zuogu
2. Huantiao (GB30)

Back Fasciitis

Ashi–Yanglingquan (GB34)

For this pair of points, acupoint injection is more effective than acupuncture. Performing acupuncture alone can be effective.

Case: Mr. Chen, a 50-year-old man, suffered from left upper back pain for 1 month. He found it difficult to bend and raise his right arm. He had tenderness on his back with stiff muscular fasciae. His tongue was red with white fur and a small string-like pulse. We diagnosed him with back fasciitis. Considering that the lung is beneath the affected area, we performed acupuncture first. However, it was ineffective. We then switched to acupoint injection. After two sessions of treatment, the disease was cured.

Fasciitis can be caused by overwork, injury, exogenous diseases, and emotional disorders. In this disease, Qi and blood flow are stagnated, liver blood is deficient, and channels lack nourishment. We normally select Danggui (Chinese angelica) injection for this treatment. Danggui has a pungent and bitter taste. As bitterness can cause purgation and pungency can cause dispersing, Danggui can activate blood flow. It is fragrant and warm; therefore, it can activate Qi, resolve stagnation, and stop pain. Danggui enters the liver channel. The tendons and ligament are governed by the liver and nourished by blood. If liver blood is deficient, tendons and ligaments can contract. Danggui injection can relieve blood stagnation. The Yanglingquan (GB34) is the convergence of the tendons and the He-Sea point on the foot Shaoyang. It can relieve muscle rigidity, activate collaterals, and disperse fire of the liver and gallbladder. Selecting this pair of points can active Qi, disperse stagnation, nourish tendons, and eliminate pathogenic factors.

Back Fasciitis

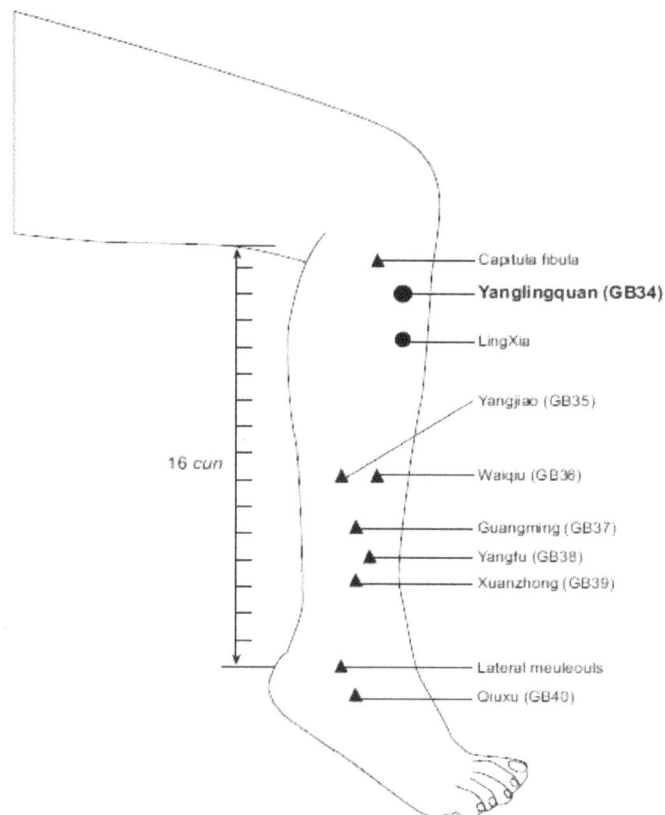

Knee Arthritis
Xinxi (11.09)–Xiji

Xiji is located 1 *cun* above and 0.5 *cun* inside the Xuehai (SP10).

Needling technique: Insert a filiform needle perpendicularly and quickly. After the needle touches the femur, lift the needle slightly and insert it upward 1 *cun* further along the femur. The needle is in the appropriate place when you feel resistance. This point is approximately 2–2.5 *cun* deep. Leave the needle in place for 30 min.

We have used this pair of points for treating knee pain in many cases. As long as the point is properly located, this method can be effective.

[Experience]: We used this pair of points to treat knee arthritis in a sergeant from California. We received an award because of the treatment. We also used this pair of points to successfully treat arthritis in foreign residents.

Knee Arthritis

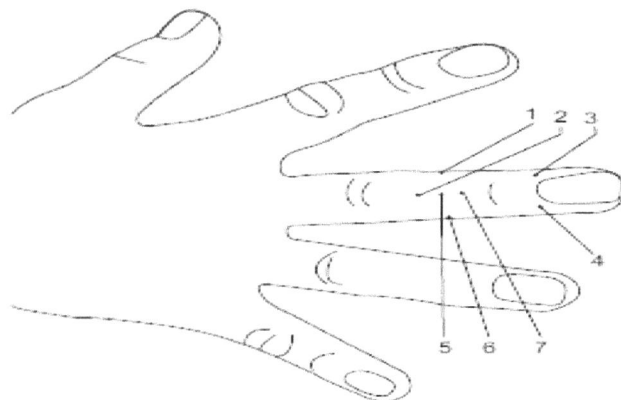

1. Xinxi (11.09)
2. Feixin (11.11)
3. Xilingyi
4. Xilinger
5. Feixin (11.11)
6. Xinxi (11.09)
7. Feixin (11.11)

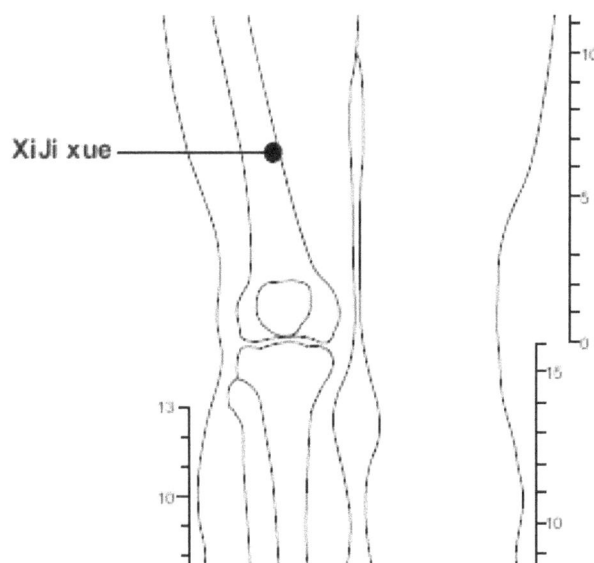

XiJi xue

Tuberculosis of the Knee

Tuberculosis of the Knee

The treatment of crane-like arthrosis was recorded by Sun Simiao during the Tang Dynasty (618–907 A.D.) in his book Qianjin Yaofang. He thought that the Xiaxi (GB43) and the Xiyangguan (GB33) could be used for treating diseases outside the knee. In the Song Dynasty (960–1279 A.D.), Wang Zhizhong summarized in his Zhenjiu Zishengjing Xitong that the Ququan (LR8) and the Xiyangguan (GB33) can be used for treating pain inside the knee.

Weizhong (BL40)–Yangjiao (GB35)

Bloodletting therapy is performed. Select the Weizhong (BL40) and the Yangjiao (GB35). After sterilization, prick the vein at these two points with three-edged needles. Let approximately 10 ml of blood flow out. After the bleeding stops, perform cupping therapy. After the therapy, sterilize the area with 2% iodine on a cotton ball.

Case: Ms. Wang, a 21-year-old woman, injured her right knee while playing volleyball 3 months ago. Her knee had swollen and burned. She found it difficult to walk. After knee aspiration and anti-inflammation treatment, the symptoms did not improve.

Examination: She had a sad-looking face and emaciated body. Her right leg was half bent. The range of motion was approximately 10°. Her knee was swollen, fusiform, tender, and warm. Fluctuation could be felt. The quadriceps were atrophic. Lymph nodes in the groin were enlarged. A blood test showed a white blood cell count of 210×10^9/L, neutrophil levels of 0.64, lymphocyte levels of 0.18, and erythrocyte sedimentation rate of 65 mm/h. X-ray showed bone destruction on the articular surface. We diagnosed right knee tuberculosis complicated with mixed infection in the patient.

After one session of treatment, the right knee swelling and pain were relieved. The range of motion was approximately 30°. White blood cell counts was 1.2×10^9/L. After three sessions of treatment, right knee swelling and pain was drastically reduced. The enlarged lymph nodes in the groin disappeared. She could extend her right leg.

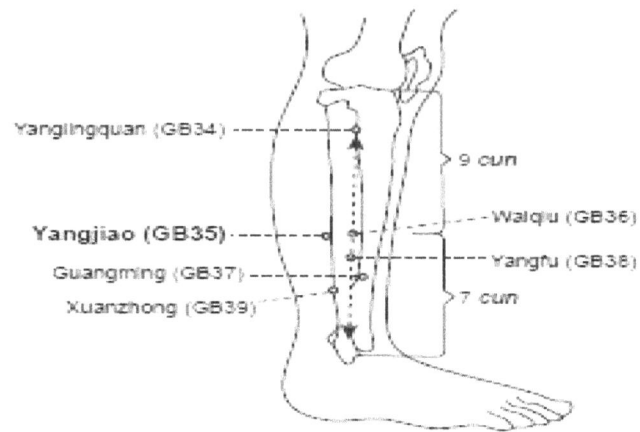

Yanglingquan (GB34)
9 cun
Waiqiu (GB36)
Yangjiao (GB35)
Yangfu (GB38)
Guangming (GB37)
Xuanzhong (GB39)
7 cun

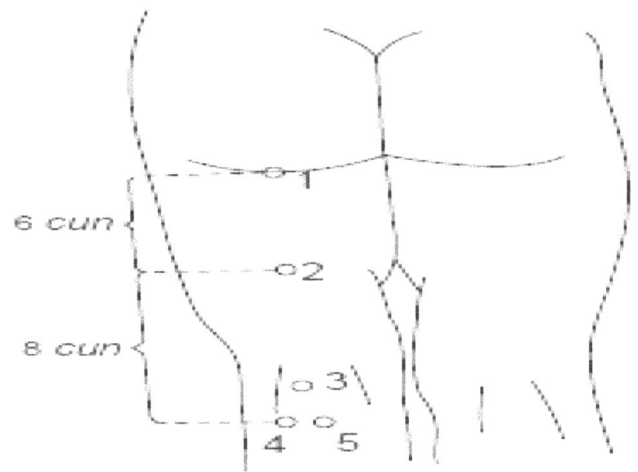

6 cun
8 cun

1. Chengfu (BL36)
2. Yinmen (BL37)
3. Fuxi (BL38)
4. Weiyang (BL39)
5. Weizhong (BL40)

Chondromalacia Patellae

Chondromalacia Patellae

Xuehai (SP10)–Liangqiu (ST34)

Acupuncture is performed. Select the Xuehai (SP10) and the Liangqiu (ST34). Sterilize the points with a tincture of iodine and alcohol. Insert needles deeply into the points with the needle tips touching the femur. The needle insertion sensation will spread to the knee. Next, perform vibration and Qi-activating needling for 1–3 min. If the patient feels aching, distension, or warmth in the knee, remove the needles and press the site.

This method was used for treat 35 cases of chondromalacia patellae. Usually, patients felt relaxation in the knees after the needles were removed. On an average, symptoms disappeared after eight sessions of treatment. After the symptoms disappeared, tenderness and friction pain in the knee also disappeared. The friction sensation under the patellae, however, often persisted.

This disease belongs to impediment syndrome (bi syndrome) in TCM. Bi syndrome is caused by blockage. Being weak, catching a cold, dampness, and Qi and blood stagnation in the knee are the original causes. Thus, treatment should focus on regulating and nourishing Qi and blood, eliminating bi, and unblocking channels. This pair of points is on the spleen and stomach channels, respectively. They can be used for nourishing the origin of Qi, reinforcing blood, and eliminating bi. The needling technique, in which needles are inserted deeply, is mainly used for treating bone bi. It was called as the short needling technique in ancient times. The goal of vibration and Qi-activating needling is to perform sufficient stimulation within the patient's tolerance limits.

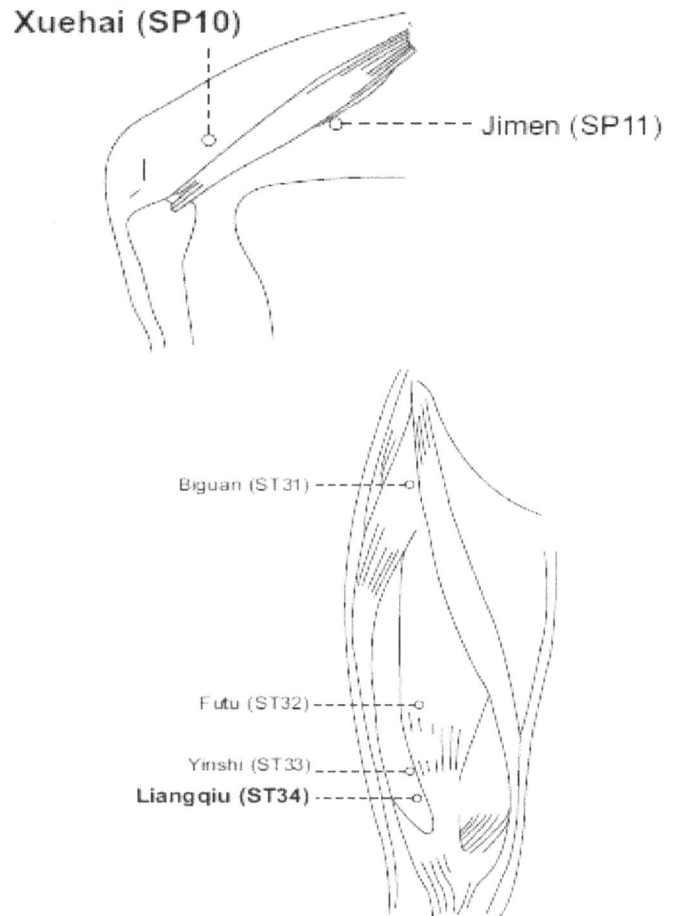

Xuehai (SP10)
Jimen (SP11)
Biguan (ST31)
Futu (ST32)
Yinshi (ST33)
Liangqiu (ST34)

Meniscus Injury

Meniscus Injury

Weizhong (BL40)–Yanglingquan (GB34)

Bloodletting therapy is performed. Select the Yanglingquan (GB34) on the affected side. Prick the points with three-edged needles to let some blood flow out. Routine sterilization is performed.

Case: Gary, a 34-year-old Mexican guard, injured his left knee after slipping and falling while jogging 3 months ago. His knee was swollen and painful. He found it difficult to walk.

When he came to our clinic, his left leg was half bent. His left knee had tenderness and was swollen. The quadriceps and gastrocnemius were slightly atrophic. He was diagnosed with meniscus injury. We used this method and prescribed *Gancao Fuzi* decoction (one decoction daily) for treatment. After half a month, he came for a second appointment. This time, his left knee felt relaxed and could bend. The pain was relieved. After another half month (at the third appointment), the pain in his knee had disappeared. We prescribed *Jingui Shenqi* pills (5 g), twice daily to regulate his Yang Qi. We asked him to take the pills for 1 month. At the 6-month follow-up, the symptoms had not recurred.

Weizhong (BL40) is the He-Sea point on the foot Taiyang bladder channel. Yanglingquan (GB34) is the He-Sea point on the foot Shaoyang gallbladder channel and the convergence of tendons. When the meniscus is injured, there will be veins showing near the Weizhong (BL40) and the Yanglingquan (GB34). Combined with herbal medicine, pricking these points to let some blood flow out is particularly effective in patients who have not been cured after long-term treatment and suffer from coagulated cold.

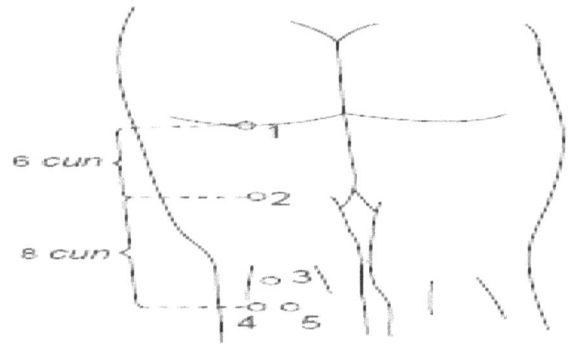

1. Chengfu (BL36)
2. Yinmen (BL37)
3. Fuxi (BL38)
4. Weiyang (BL39)
5. Weizhong (BL40)

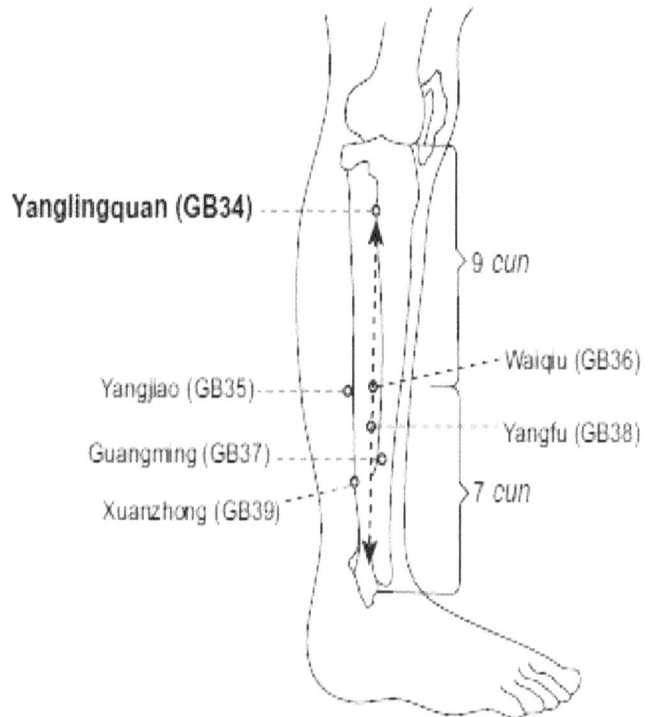

Hyperosteogeny at Heel

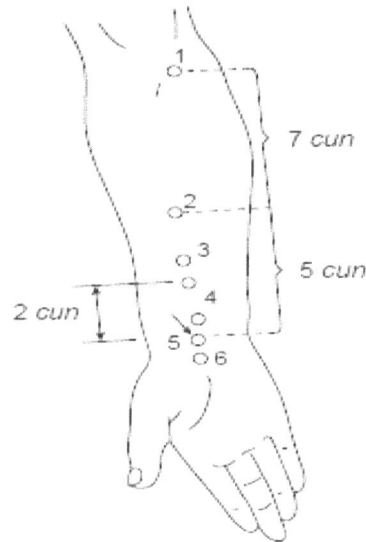

Hyperosteogeny at Heel

Zugen (Hand point)–Baihui (GV20)

Zugen: A hand point located 0.8 *cun* beneath the Daling (PC7). Acupuncture is performed. After routine sterilization, insert a needle measuring (0.45–0.38 mm) * (15–25 mm) into the Zugen on the unaffected side. After the needle penetrates the skin, insert it upward obliquely. Dong-Qi needling is performed. Leave the needles in place for 30 min. One session of treatment includes acupuncture for 15 consecutive days. Start another session after a 7-day interval.

This method can be used for treating hyperosteogeny at the heel as well as heel pain caused by injury. It is immediately effective. Zugen is different from Mr. Dong's extra points Guguan (22.24) and Muguan (22.26). Besides Dong's extra points, practitioners have to learn more about these points. As Dong's extra points differ from traditional points, practitioners must know the differences when using these points. Only when these points are learned and well differentiated, can they be used effectively.

7 cun

5 cun

2 cun

1. Quze (PC3)
2. Ximen (PC4)
3. Jianshi (PC5)
4. Neiguan (PC6)
5. Daling (PC7)
6. Zugen

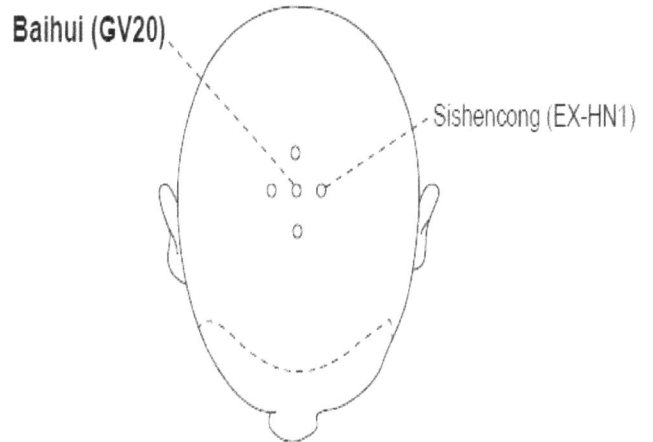

Baihui (GV20)

Sishencong (EX-HN1)

Taiyuan (LU9)–Yuji (LU10)

Acupuncture is performed. After routine sterilization, insert needles into these points on the affected side at 0.5–0.8 *cun* deep. Leave the needles in place for 20–30 min. Perform acupuncture once every other day.

We have used this method for treating sequelae of fracture in one case. It was cured after six sessions of treatment.

Case: Datian, a 23-year-old housewife, developed a fracture of the lower radius. After routine treatment over 3 months, the fracture healed. However, pain, swelling, and numbness in the wrist and elbow persisted. She had a normal tongue and floating and tight pulse. She often had aversion to cold with fever, which are symptoms of exterior cold damp syndrome. We diagnosed sequelae of fracture in the patient and treated her with this method combined with three doses of *Mahuang Jiazhu* decoction. After two sessions of treatment, the symptoms disappeared. To consolidate the effectiveness, we prescribed five doses of *Huoluo Xiaoling* Pills. The disease was cured after 4 months.

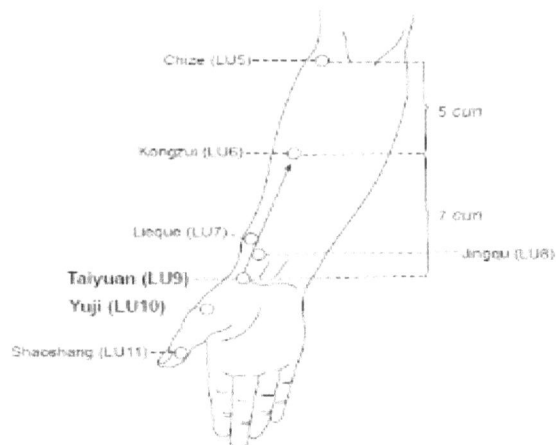

Chapter Four

Internal Diseases

Section One

Diseases of the Cardiovascular System

Palpitation

Formula One: Xinmen (33.12)–Sihuazhong (77.09)

Acupuncture and bloodletting are performed. First, insert a needle into the Xinmen (33.12) at 1.5 *cun* deep. Insert it upward along the bone. Leave the needle in place for 15–20 min without manipulation. Then, prick the Sihuazhong (77.09) and let the blood flow out. In most patients with angina pectoris, the pain will stop after treatment. Patients can breathe properly.

Formula Two: Xindian (hand point)–Zhiyang (GV9)

Acupuncture is performed, regardless of the needle technique.

Xindian: An extra point located at the palmar surface of the middle finger, midpoint of the distal finger crease.

Case: Ms. Chuanqi, a 54-year-old housewife, developed heart disease 3 years ago. Her symptoms became worse when she overworked. Her heart and respiratory rates became irregular and were accompanied by chest pain. She had a rapid weak pulse and red tongue without fur. After treatment with Formula One, she could breathe properly. Chest pain did not recur. After five more sessions of treatment, chest tightness and breathing trouble were largely relieved.

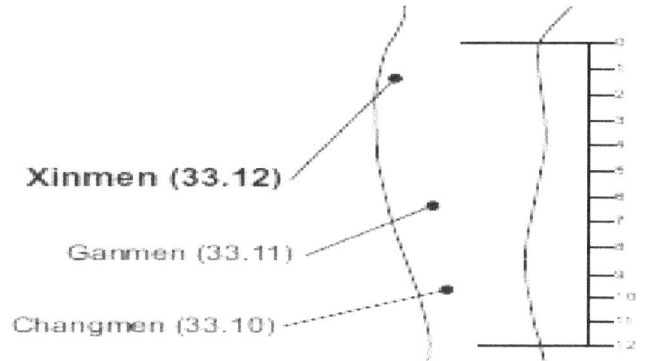

Xinmen (33.12)
Ganmen (33.11)
Changmen (33.10)

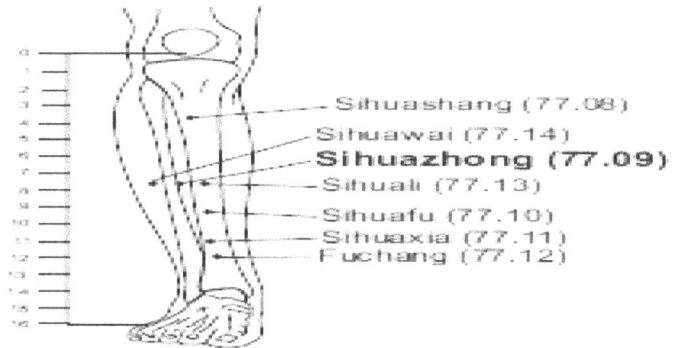

Sihuashang (77.08)
Sihuawai (77.14)
Sihuazhong (77.09)
Sihuali (77.13)
Sihuafu (77.10)
Sihuaxia (77.11)
Fuchang (77.12)

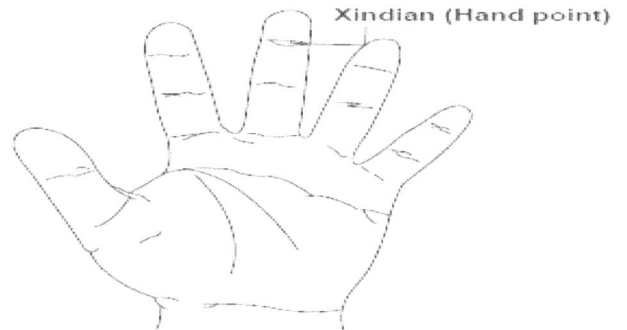

Xindian (Hand point)

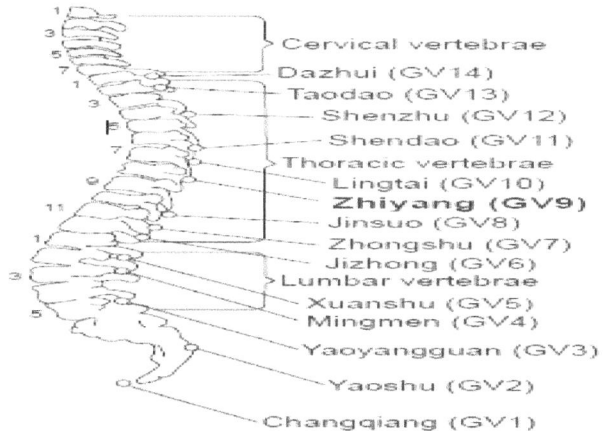

Cervical vertebrae
Dazhui (GV14)
Taodao (GV13)
Shenzhu (GV12)
Shendao (GV11)
Thoracic vertebrae
Lingtai (GV10)
Zhiyang (GV9)
Jinsuo (GV8)
Zhongshu (GV7)
Jizhong (GV6)
Lumbar vertebrae
Xuanshu (GV5)
Mingmen (GV4)
Yaoyangguan (GV3)
Yaoshu (GV2)
Changqiang (GV1)

Arrhythmia

Arrhythmia refers to a heartbeat that is too rapid, too slow, or irregular, including abnormality in the natural pacemaker and/or disorder of conduction. Symptoms include palpitations, dizziness, chest tightness, nausea, pale complexion, cold sweating, and even fainting. When the heart beats too rapidly, i.e., >100 beats/min, it is called tachycardia. When the heart beats too slowly, i.e., <60 beats/min, it is called bradycardia. When the heart beats rapidly at one time and slowly at another, it is called an irregular heart rate (arrhythmia). In the theory of traditional Chinese medicine, arrhythmia comprises fright palpitation, severe palpitation, and fainting.

Renying (ST9)–Neiguan (PC6)

Acupuncture is performed. Filiform needles are used. Select points on both sides. Insert a needle inward obliquely into the Renying (ST9) at 1–1.5 *cun* deep. The needle should be pulsatile with the pulse, regardless of the needle technique. Insert a needle into the Neiguan (PC6) perpendicularly at 0.5 *cun* deep, performing the sparrow-pecking needle technique. The needle pricking sensation will spread to the middle finger and elbow.

Case: A 33-year-old woman working at a restaurant developed palpitations, shortness of breath, and sweating when quarreling with others. When she visited our clinic, her heart rate was 187 beats/min. Her heart rhythm was regular. Blood pressure was 14.7/9.3 KPa (110/70 mm Hg). She was diagnosed with paroxysmal supraventricular tachycardia complicated with intraventricular aberrant conduction based on her electrocardiogram (ECG) results. We used this pair of points to treat her. After treatment, her heart rate became 107 beats/min with a regular rhythm.

The Renying (ST9) is at the same level as the laryngeal prominence. As the carotid artery and many nerves are present at this point, it is sensitive. Stimulation of the Renying (ST9) can regulate the heart rhythm through nerve and channel conduction. The Neiguan (PC6) is an important point for treating diseases of the heart and chest. Treatment with a combination of these two points can be easily effective. Effectiveness of this treatment depends on locating the points properly, using the proper needle technique, right diagnosis, and achieving the needle pricking sensation. If the points are located properly and the right needle technique is used, the greater distension felt on the site during the needle pricking sensation is better. This can also help the heart rhythm to recover sooner. If arrhythmia is a deficiency syndrome caused by fright and overwork, the Shenmen (HT7) and Sanyinjiao (SP6) can be selected with the twisting reinforcing needle technique. If arrhythmia is caused by emotional distress and annoyance, the Taichong (LR3) can be selected with the lift-thrust reducing needle technique.

Arrhythmia

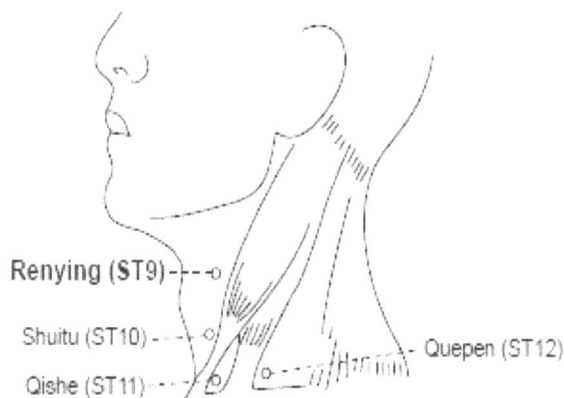

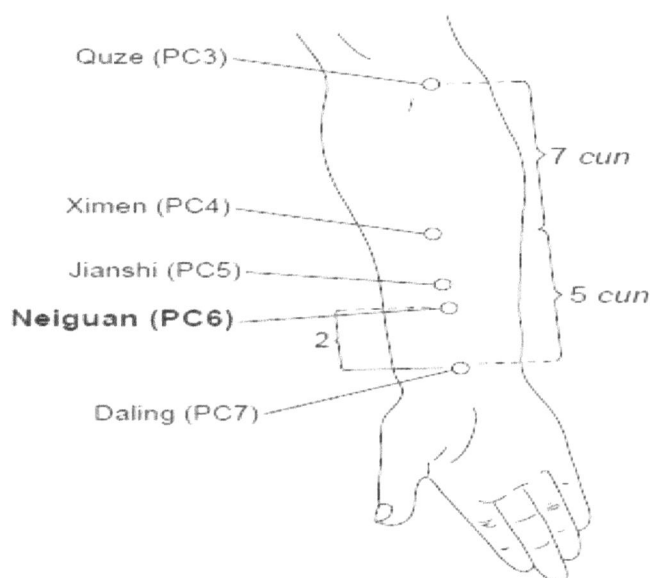

Coronary Atherosclerotic Heart Disease and Angina Pectoris

Treatment of coronary heart disease with acupuncture is recorded in many ancient books. It was first recorded in Neijing. The disease was termed as heart pain and was said to be associated with the five viscera in Neijing. There are four signs and treatments according to Lingshu Juebing: "True heart pain with cold limbs, which is observed as bloating, chest tightness, and severe heart pain, is true heart pain with cold limbs caused by stomach disease. It can be treated by acupuncture on the Dadu (SP2) and Taibai (SP3)." "True heart pain with cold limbs, which is felt as the heart being pricked by a stabber and severe heart pain, is true heart pain with cold limbs caused by spleen disease, and it can be treated by acupuncture on the Rangu (KI2) and Taixi (KI3)." "True heart pain with cold limbs, which is observed as a blue complexion and shortness of breath, is true heart pain with cold limbs caused by liver disease, and it can be treated by acupuncture on the Xingjian (LR2) and Taichong (LR3)." "True heart pain with cold limbs, which is normal when lying and becomes worse when moving without causing complexion changes, is true heart pain with cold limbs caused by lung disease, and it can be treated by acupuncture on the Yuji (LU10) and Taiyuan (LU9)."

Thoracic Cavity Area (Scalp Acupuncture)–Sensory Area (Scalp Acupuncture)

Prime Meridian

There are two prime meridians: antero-posterior midline and eyebrow occiput line. The antero-posterior midline is the line connecting the glabellum with the lower border of the external occipital protuberance. The eyebrow occiput line is the line connecting the mid-point of the upper border of the eyebrow with the tip of the external occipital protuberance. The stimulation areas of scalp acupuncture comprise 13 lines.

Thoracic cavity area (scalp acupuncture): A 4-cm long line parallel to the antero-posterior midline, with its midpoint at the anterior hairline, midway between the line above the pupil of the eye and the midline.

Coronary Atherosclerotic

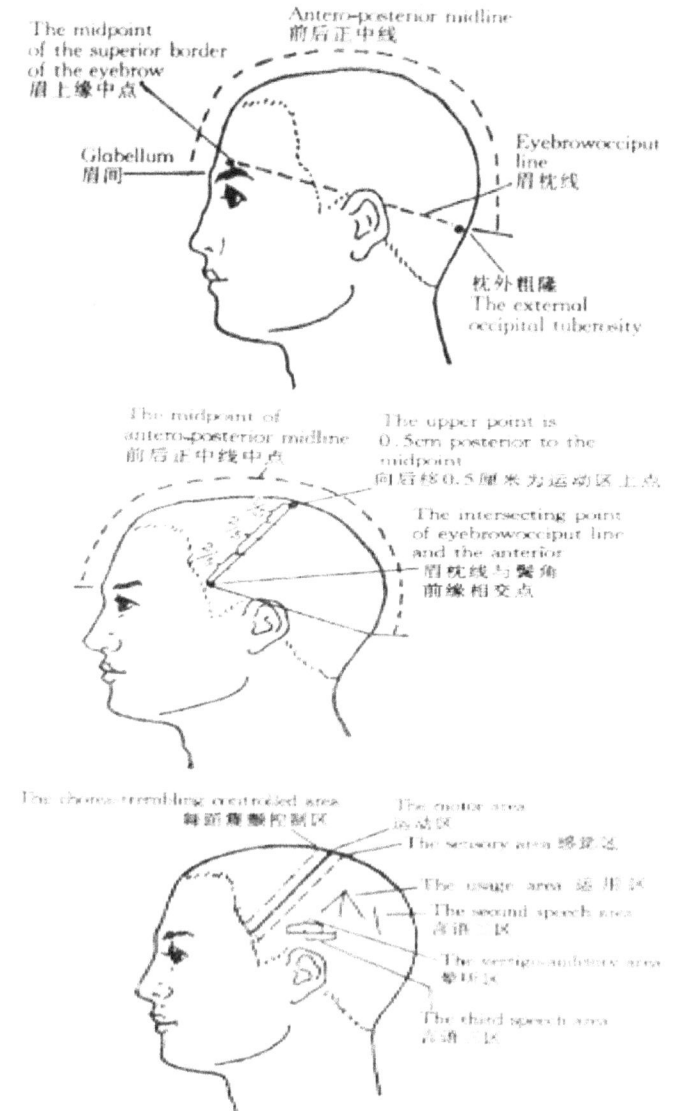

61

Coronary Atherosclerotic Heart Disease and Angina Pectoris

Sensory area (scalp acupuncture): A line parallel to and 1.5 cm posterior to the motor area (Location of the motor area: the upper point is 0.5 cm posterior to the midpoint of the antero-posterior midline and the lower point is the intersecting point of the eyebrow occiput line and the anterior border of the corner of the temporal hairline.) The upper 1/5 of the line is the sensory area for the lower limbs, head, and trunk; the middle 2/5 of the line is the sensory area for the upper limbs; and the lower 2/5 of the line the sensory area for the face.

Scalp acupuncture is performed. After routine sterilization, insert the needles quickly and twist them, making the needle pricking sensation spread to the heart.

Coronary Atherosclerotic Heart Disease and Angina Pectoris

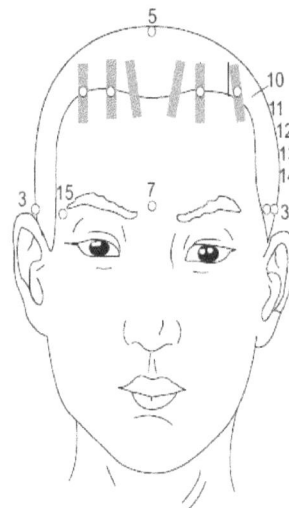

1. Gastric Area
2. Hepatocystic Area
3. Midpoint of the Vertigo-Auditory Area
4. Lower point of the Motor Area
5. Upper Point of the Vasomotor Area
6. Midline of the forehead
7. Glabella
8. Thoracic Area
9. Reproductive Area
10. Intestine Area
11. Vasomotor Area
12. Chorea-Tremor Control Area
13. Motor Area
14. Sensory Area
15. (Intersecting point of the eyebrow-occipital line and the anterior border of the temple)

Myocardial Infarction

Myocardial infarction is caused by blockage of the coronary artery, which results in ischemic necrosis of the myocardium. Symptoms include severe and persistent chest pain, shock, fever, increased white blood cell counts, increased ESR, increased serum myocardial enzyme levels, and ECG changes. In the theory of traditional Chinese medicine, myocardial infarction comprises true heart pain and true heart pain with cold limbs.

Danzhong (CV17)–Lingdao (HT4)

Acupuncture is performed. Insert a needle 2.5–2.8 *cun* deep into the Danzhong (CV17) along the skin and penetrate the needle through the Jiuwei (CV15). Perform moderate-to-strong stimulation. Press and knead the Lingdao (HT4) for 1.5 min. Subsequently, press the point vigorously for 2 min. Afterward, knead the point slightly for 1.5 min.

Myocardial Infarction

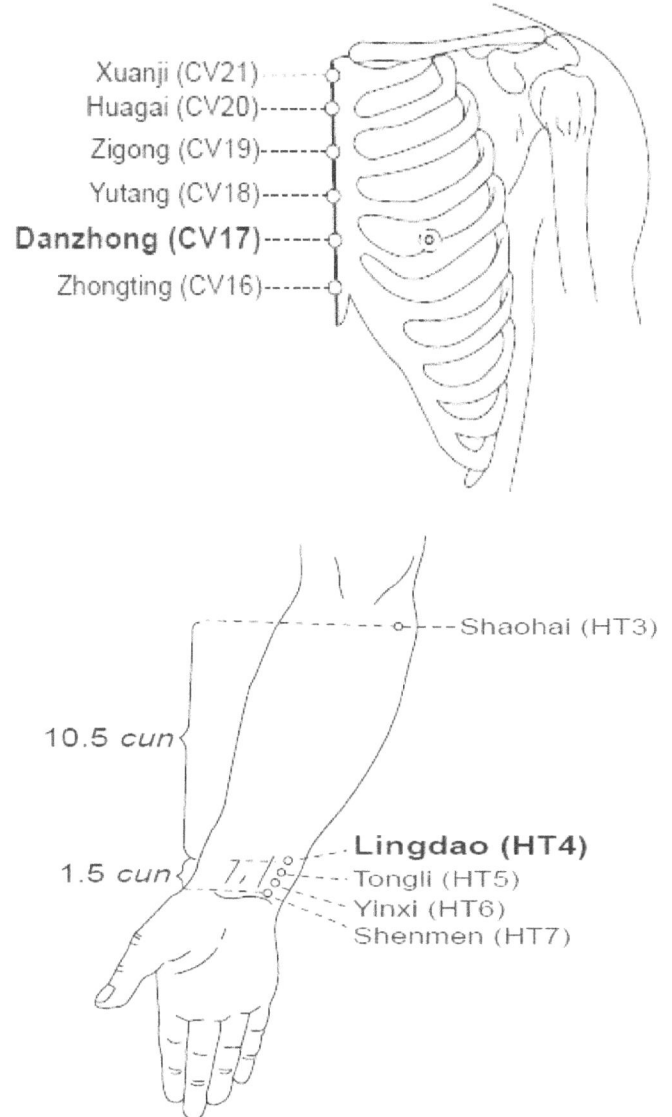

63

Hypertension

Hypertension refers to increased pressure in the blood vessels. In the theory of traditional Chinese medicine, hypertension comprises dizziness and headache. Signs and symptoms include blood pressure > 18.7/12.0 KPa (140/90 mm Hg), dizziness, headache, palpitation, insomnia, tinnitus, vexation, memory loss, flush, and extremity numbness.

Formula One: Gandanqu (eye point)

Insert filiform needles into this area. After achieving the needle pricking sensation, leave the needles in place for 15 min.

Formula Two: Jianjing (GB21)–Xueya

Xueya: An extra point located 2 *cun* lateral to the C6 spinous process. Acupuncture is performed. When inserting the needles into the Xueya, the tips of the needles should be upward at 1–2 *cun* deep. The Jianjing (GB21) should be carefully inserted. The needles should be <2 *cun* deep.

Case: Mr. Wang, a 45-year-old man, suffered from hypertension for 5 years and was a smoker and drinker. His blood pressure was often 21.3–25.3/13.3–14.6 KPa. He experienced dizziness and headache, irritable mood, tinnitus, vexation, chest tightness, insomnia, a bitter taste in his mouth, bad breath, and right extremity numbness. He often took western medicine to control his blood pressure. However, the symptoms became worse; therefore, he visited our clinic for treatment. On examination, it was observed that he had a red tongue with ecchymosis on the sides and stagnated veins under his tongue. His tongue was thin, white, and slightly yellow. He had a string-like, slippery, and rapid pulse. The diagnosis was upper hyperactivity of the liver Yang and blood stagnation, which should be treated by suppressing hyperactive liver, subsiding the Yang, activating blood circulation, and resolving stasis. We treated him with this method. On the 2nd day, his blood pressure reduced to 21.3/12.8 KPa. Dizziness and irritability were relieved. After 2 weeks of this treatment combined with needle insertion at the Neiguan (PC6) with the reducing-twirling technique, his blood pressure reduced to 18.6/10.7 KPa. To consolidate this effect, we also administered herbal medicine. Treatment was effective.

Hypertension

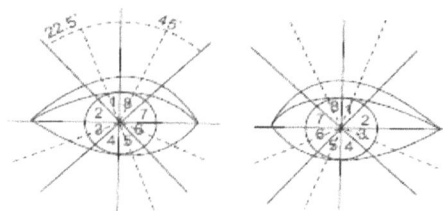

Right eye   **Left eye**

1. Shen Pangguang (kidney and bladder)
2. Shangjiao (Upper Energizer)
3. **Gandan (liver and gallbladder)**
4. Zhongjiao (Middle Energizer)
5. Xin Xiaochang (heart and small intestine)
6. Piwei (spleen and stomach)
7. Xiajiao (Lower Energizer)
8. Fei Dachang (lung and large intestine)

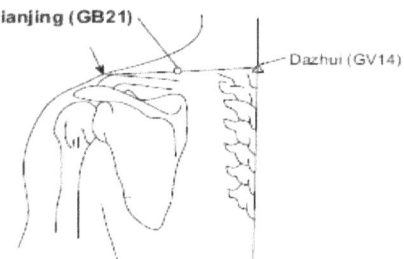

Jianjing (GB21)

Dazhui (GV14)

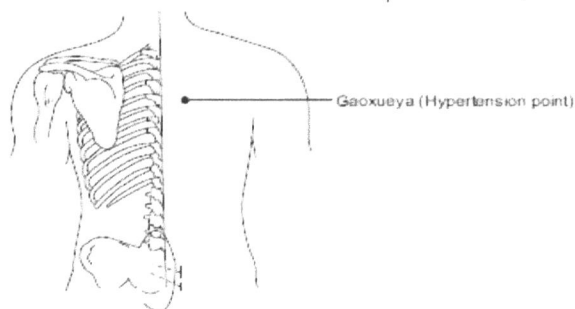

Gaoxueya (Hypertension point)

Hypertension

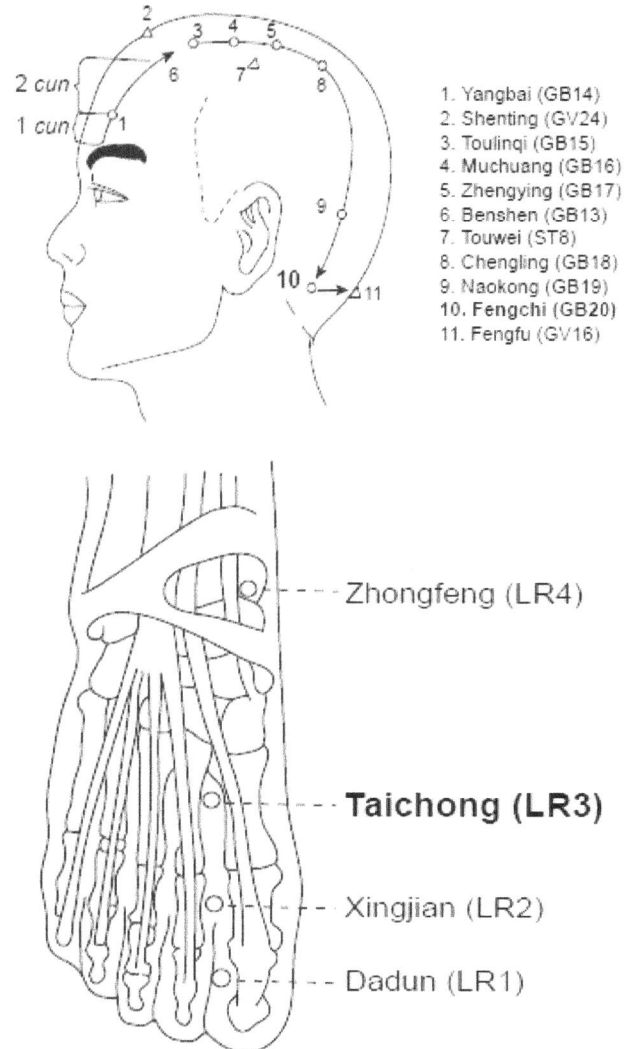

Hypertension

Formula Three: Fengchi (GB20)–Taichong (LR3)

Perform bloodletting therapy on the Fengchi (GB20) and acupuncture on the Taichong (LR3) with the tip of needle pointing upward. Perform the reducing needle technique.

We use Formula Three for treating dizziness and headaches caused by hypertension. It is immediately effective and patients are satisfied with the treatment.

1. Yangbai (GB14)
2. Shenting (GV24)
3. Toulinqi (GB15)
4. Muchuang (GB16)
5. Zhengying (GB17)
6. Benshen (GB13)
7. Touwei (ST8)
8. Chengling (GB18)
9. Naokong (GB19)
10. Fengchi (GB20)
11. Fengfu (GV16)

Zhongfeng (LR4)

Taichong (LR3)

Xingjian (LR2)

Dadun (LR1)

Hypotension

Hypotension is a common disease. For adults, a normal systolic blood pressure is 12–18.7 KPa (90–140 mm Hg). A normal diastolic blood pressure is 8–12 KPa (60–90 mm Hg). If systolic pressure is <12.0 Kpa or if diastolic pressure is <8.0 Kpa, it is termed as hypotension or low blood pressure. Hypotension can be divided into acute and chronic. Acute hypotension is usually accompanied by fainting or shock. Chronic hypotension often has no symptoms. However, a few patients have reported dizziness, vertigo, weakness, and coldness in the extremities. Chronic hypotension is usually caused by hormonal disorders, chronic consumptive disease, malnutrition, or cardiovascular diseases. In the theory of traditional Chinese medicine, hypotension comprises insufficiency and vertigo.

Yangchi (TE4)–Baihui (GV20)

Acupuncture is performed. At the Baihui (GV20), perform strong stimulation with the uniform reinforcing-reducing needle technique. At the Yangchi (TE4), if proper needle technique is used, the treatment can be immediately effective.

Case: Ms. Li, a 29-year-old woman, suffered from pain, which was more severe in the lower extremities, for many years. The pain was accompanied by tinnitus, vertigo, sweating from the head, cold hands and feet, and frequent urination. Her blood pressure was 12.0/8.0 KPa (90/60 mm Hg). After one session of treatment, her blood pressure increased to 13.6/9.3 KPa (102/70 mm Hg).

Hypotension

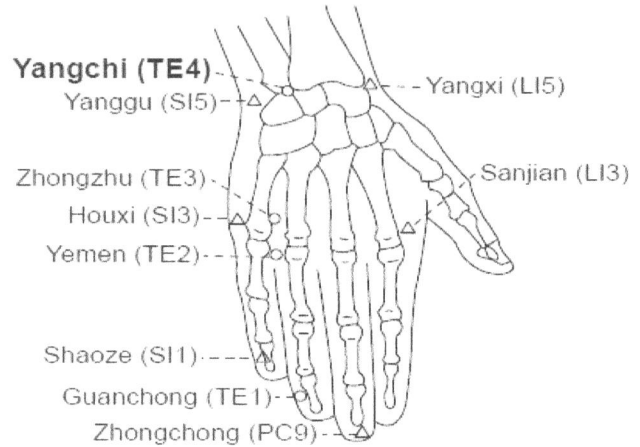

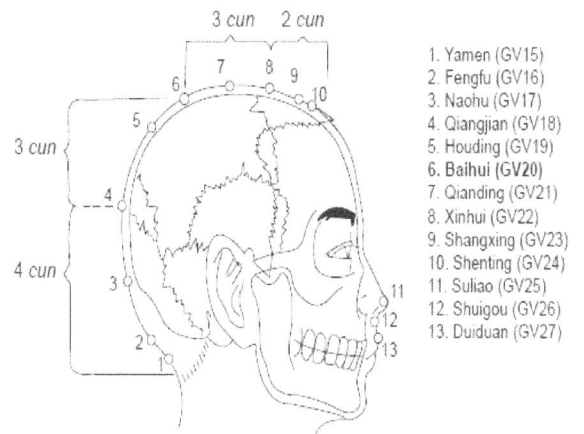

1. Yamen (GV15)
2. Fengfu (GV16)
3. Naohu (GV17)
4. Qiangjian (GV18)
5. Houding (GV19)
6. Baihui (GV20)
7. Qianding (GV21)
8. Xinhui (GV22)
9. Shangxing (GV23)
10. Shenting (GV24)
11. Suliao (GV25)
12. Shuigou (GV26)
13. Duiduan (GV27)

Section Two

Diseases of the Respiratory System

Cold

Formula One: Sanchasan (22.17)–Erjian (Ear point)

Perform acupuncture on the Sanchayi (22.15), Sanchaer (22.16), and Sanchasan (22.17) points, which are Dong's secret points. Combine acupuncture with bloodletting therapy on the Erjian (ear point) and veins on the back of the ears. Acupuncture on the Sanchayi (22.15), Sanchaer (22.16), and Sanchasan (22.17) should be combined with acupuncture on the assistant points. Most of Dong's students are not willing to share these secret points with their colleagues. These points can be used for treating fatigue syndromes, sprains, and generalized pain. Treatment using these points is more effective than that using Dong's three special points for cold (88.07, 88.08, and 88.09).

Formula Two: Shenmai (BL62)–Houxi (SI3)

Acupuncture is performed. Insert a needle perpendicularly into the Shenmai (BL62). Insert another needle into the Houxi (SI3) with the tip of needle penetrating through skin of the other side. Leave the needles in place for 20 min.

Case: Mr. Dachuan, a z34-year-old man, caught cold 1 day earlier. He reported a headache, pain in the neck and shoulder, runny nose, weakness of the eyelids, lack of appetite, mild sweating, and a fever of 38.6°C. The symptoms were not relieved after taking Tylroon. We treated him with this method and he was cured after treatment.

Cold

Sanchayi (22.15)
Sanchaer (22.16)
Sanchasan (22.17)

Erjian (Ear point)

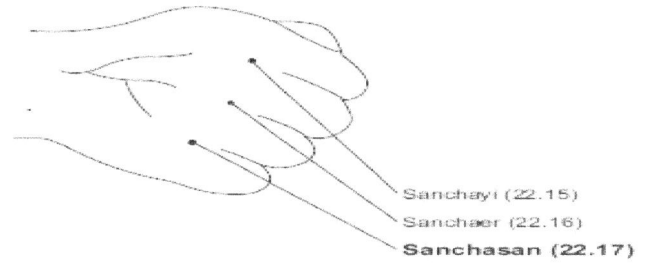

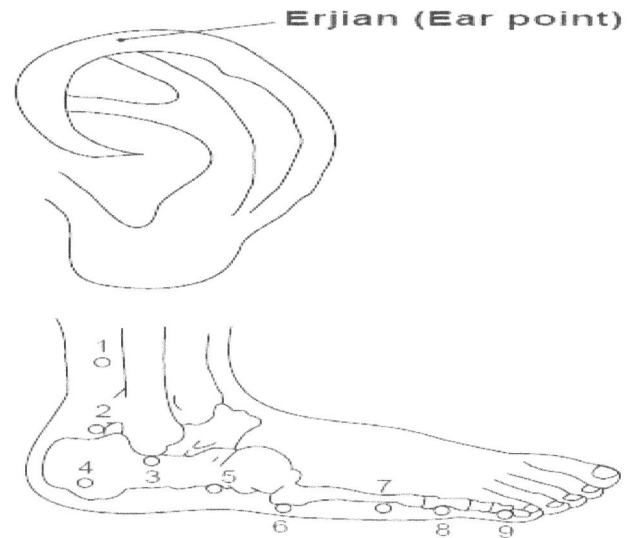

1. Fuyang (BL59)
2. Kunlun (BL60)
3. Pucan (BL61)
4. **Shenmai (BL62)**
5. Jinmen (BL63)
6. Jinggu (BL64)
7. Shugu (BL65)
8. Zutonggu (BL66)
9. Zhiyin (BL67)

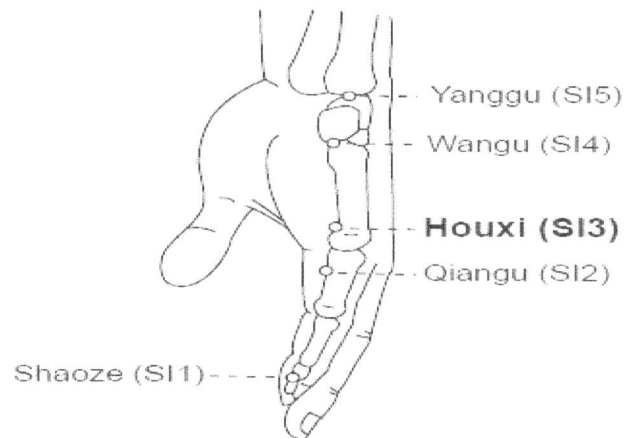

Yanggu (SI5)
Wangu (SI4)
Houxi (SI3)
Qiangu (SI2)
Shaoze (SI1)

67

Upper Respiratory Tract Infection

Upper Respiratory Tract Infection

Upper respiratory tract infection is common in children, particularly when the weather changes. The symptoms can be acute and include nasal obstruction, runny nose, sneezing, sore throat, dry mouth, high fever, diarrhea, and lack of appetite. Upper respiratory tract infection is often complicated with bronchitis and pneumonia.

Hegu (LI4)–Quchi (LI11)

Acupuncture with filiform needles is performed. Insert a needle upward and obliquely into the Hegu (LI4). Insert another needle perpendicularly into the Quchi (LI11). Perform the reducing needle technique with needle-handle flicking.

Case: Michale, a 19-year-old American man, had runny nose, fever (39°C), and red throat when he visited our clinic. There were no abnormalities with the heart, lung, or abdomen. Upper respiratory tract infection was diagnosed in the patient. He self-medicated with a pain reliever for 3 days but did not notice any improvement. We treated him with this method. One hour after treatment, his temperature decreased to 38°C. Three hours after treatment, it was 37.2°C. Four hours after treatment, it was 36.5°C. The next day, the sore throat and fever disappeared.

Hegu (LI4) and Quchi (LI11) are points on the hand Yangming channel, which is sufficient with Qi and blood. Inserting needles into these points can reduce fever and have anti-inflammatory effects.

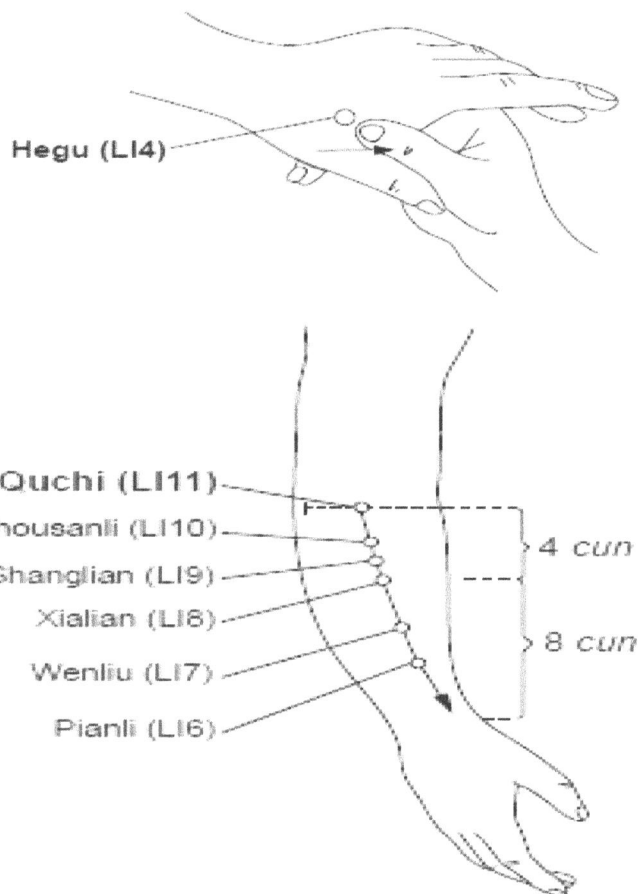

Cough

Cough

Cough is a common symptom of respiratory diseases. It may be exogenous or endogenous. Bronchitis, upper respiratory tract infection, and cold can be diagnosed as cough in the theory of traditional Chinese medicine.

Three special points for cold (88.07, 88.08, and 88.09)– Danzhong (CV17)

Acupuncture is performed without any specific needle technique. Insert a needle obliquely into Danzhong at 0.5–0.8 *cun* deep, keeping the tip along the skin. Insert needles perpendicularly or obliquely into the three special points for cold (88.07, 88.08, and 88.09). A practitioner's experience is associated with his/her knowledge of this disease.

Case: Mr. Guo, a 27-year-old salesman, was often outdoors and had a greater risk of catching cold. He suffered from cough 1 week previously without other symptoms of cold. His throat felt itchy and he kept coughing. He took western medicines, but they were not effective. We treated him with this method and he was cured after treatment.

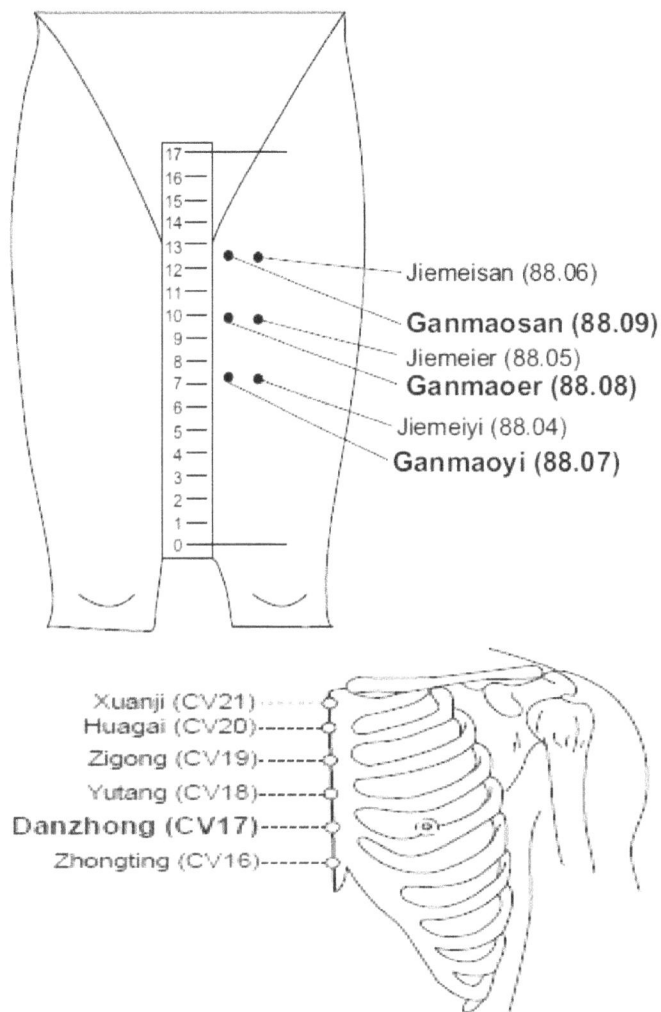

Jiemeisan (88.06)
Ganmaosan (88.09)
Jiemeier (88.05)
Ganmaoer (88.08)
Jiemeiyi (88.04)
Ganmaoyi (88.07)

Xuanji (CV21)
Huagai (CV20)
Zigong (CV19)
Yutang (CV18)
Danzhong (CV17)
Zhongting (CV16)

Bronchitis

Formula One: Tongqi–Zhichuan

Tongqi: An extra point located between the Tiantu (CV22) and Danzhong (CV17).

Zhichuan: An extra point located 0.5 *cun* lateral of the third thoracic vertebra.

Acupuncture is performed. Insert the needles approximately 1–1.5 *cun* deep, performing the reducing needle technique.

Formula Two: Taiyuan (LU9)–Sihuazhong (77.09)

Acupuncture is performed. Insert the needles 1 *cun* deep, without any specific needle technique. Leave the needles in place for 20–30 min.

Case: Christian, a 40-year-old woman, suffered from cough and wheezing for 8 years. The symptoms became worse in winter. She had cough, excessive phlegm, wheezing, chest tightness, trouble in lying flat, and shortness of breath when walking and talking. The acute attacks of chronic bronchitis often affected her work. Examination: She had moist rale in the lungs. We diagnosed her with chronic bronchitis and treated her with acupuncture combined with herbal medicine. After three sessions of treatment, she was cured.

Bronchitis

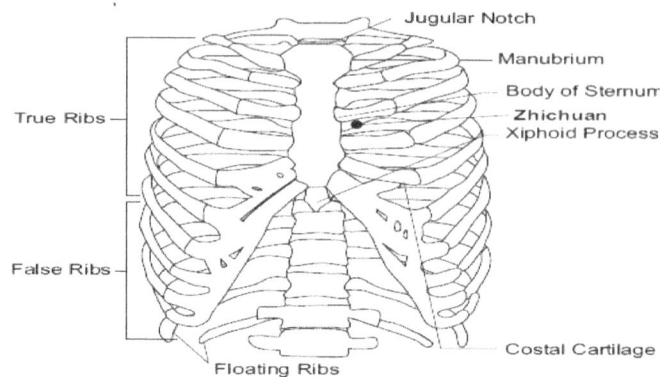

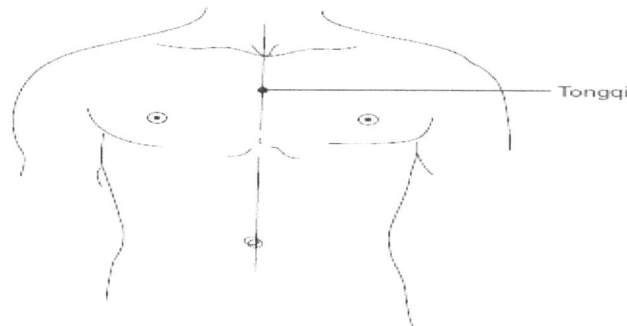

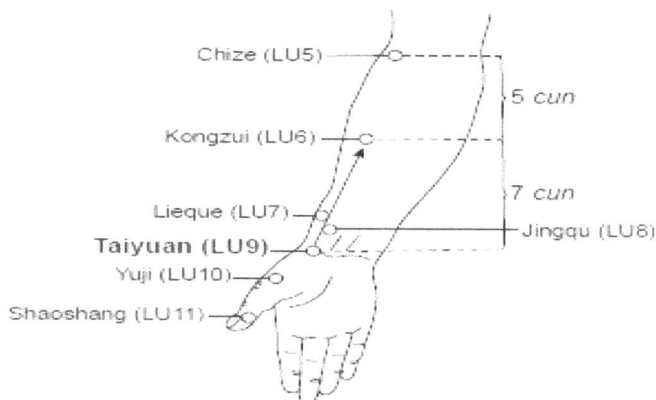

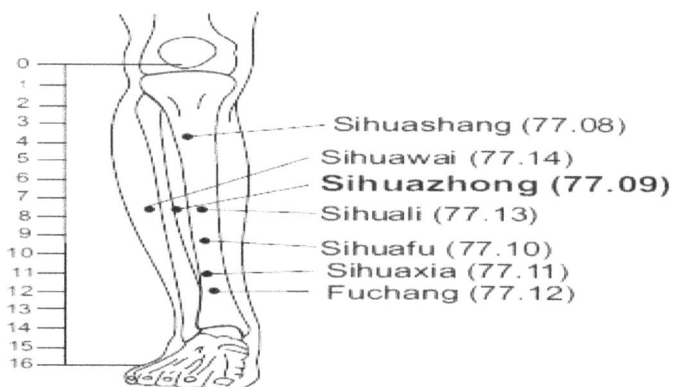

Bronchiectasis

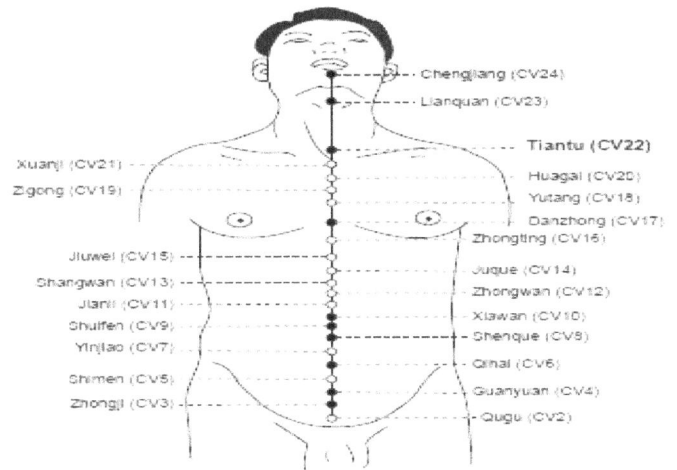

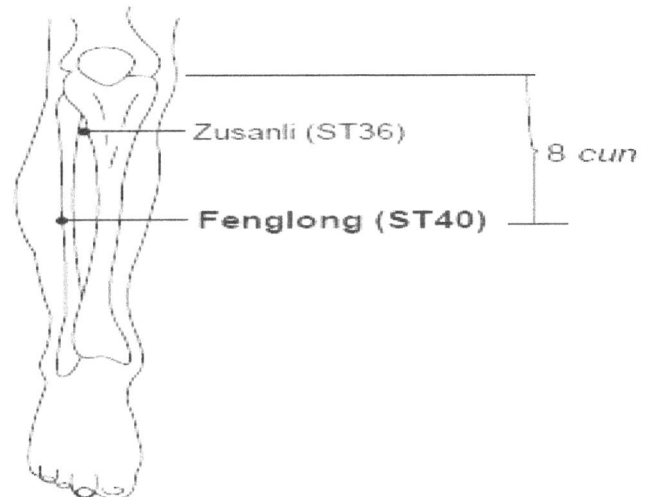

Tiantu (CV22)–Fenglong (ST40)

Acupuncture is performed with the reinforcing needle technique on the Tiantu (CV22) and the reducing needle technique on the Fenglong (ST40). Ask the patient to be seated. Press the thumb of your left hand on the Tiantu (CV22). Insert a needle obliquely into the point approximately 0.5 *cun* deep with your right hand. Twist the needle 3–4 times. Leave the needle in place for approximately 5 min before removing it. Next, insert the needles into both sides of the Fenglong (ST40) at 1 *cun* deep. Perform strong stimulation and leave the needles in place for 15 min. Bronchiectasia can be cured after 8–10 sessions of treatment with this method.

Tiantu (CV22) can be used to stop wheezing and coughing and descend adverse Qi. Bronchiectasia is often a secondary disease and is a chronic and deficiency syndrome. It should be treated with the reinforcing technique. Fenglong (ST40) is the main point for treating excessive phlegm. Performing the reducing needle technique on the Fenglong (ST40) can reduce phlegm, descend adverse Qi, and stop wheezing and coughing. These two points assist each other. Reinforcing deficiency and reducing excessiveness can be effective in reducing phlegm.

Bronchiectasis

Asthma

Asthma

Formula One: Dingchuan (EX-B1)–Yuji (LU10)

Acupuncture is performed with filiform needles. Leave the needles in place for 20–30 min, twisting the needles once every 5 min.

Formula Two: Kechuan–Zhike

Kechuan: An extra point located at the ulnar side of the second base joint, on the dorso-ventral boundary of the hand.

Zhike: An extra point located on the palmar aspect of the index finger, at the middle of the proximal phalangeal bone. For men, it is on the left hand. For women, it is on the right hand.

Acupuncture is performed. Sterilize the area and insert filiform needles measuring (0.32–0.38) * 25 mm. Twist and twirl the needles quickly to achieve the needle pricking sensation. Perform the reinforcing-reducing needle method according to respiration, until asthma and coughing stop or are relieved.

Formula Three: Shuijin (1010.20)–Dajian (11.01)

We used this method for treating asthma and achieved satisfactory results.

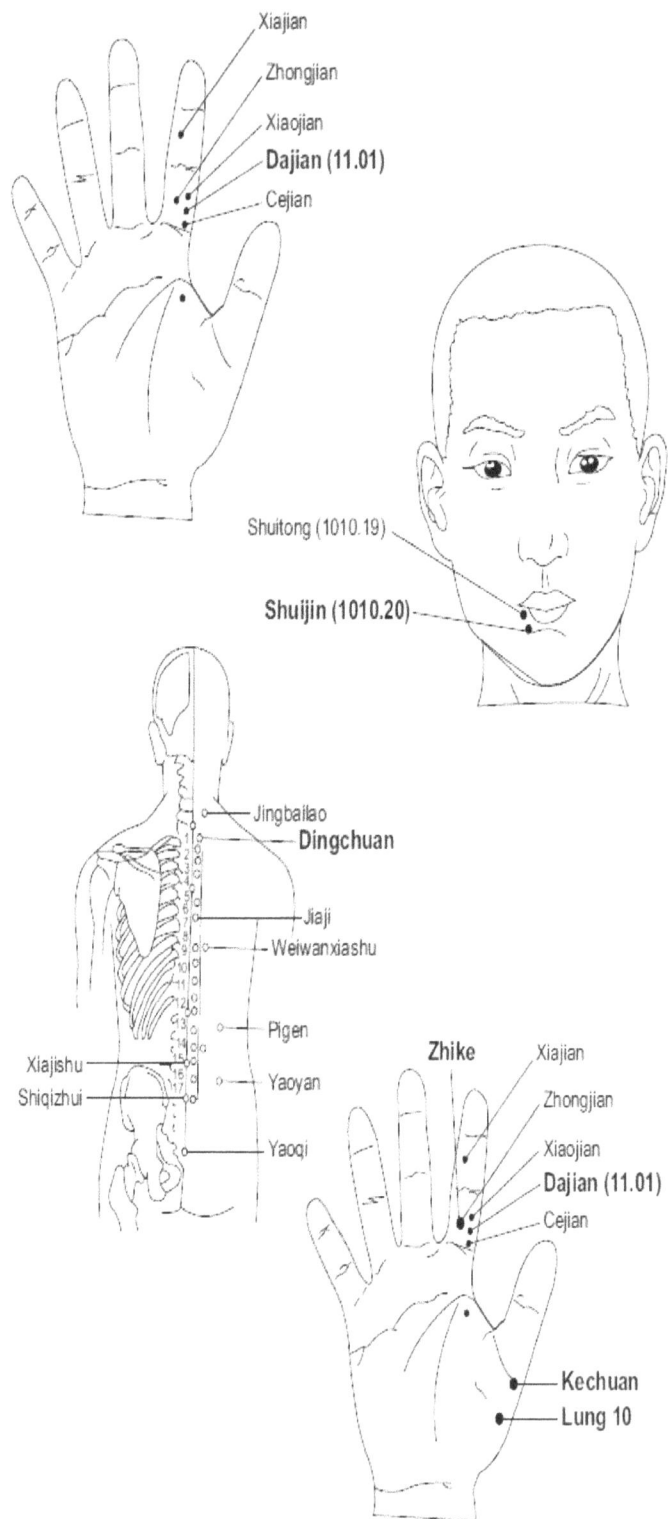

Lobar Pneumonia

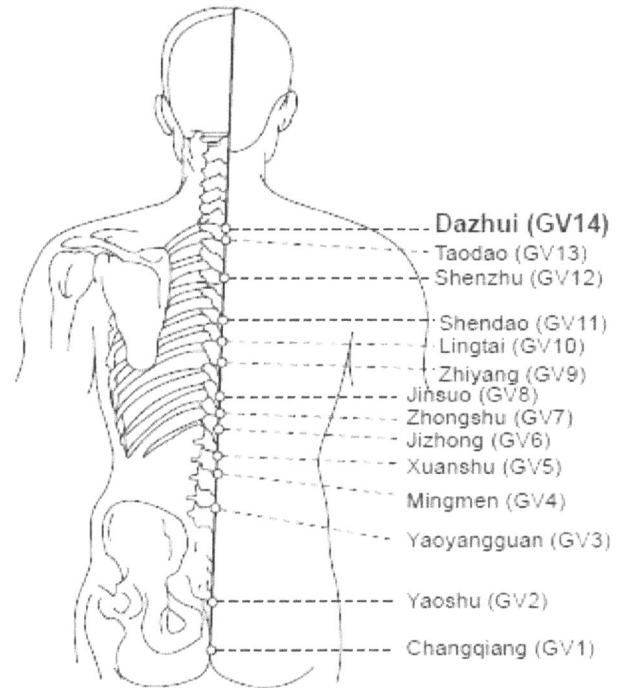

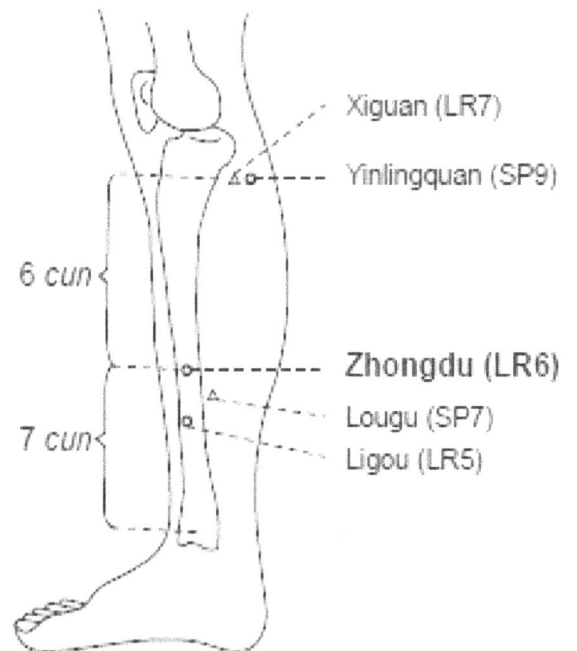

Dazhui (GV14)–Zhongdu (LR6)

Acupuncture is performed. Insert a needle obliquely into the Zhongdu (LR6) at 0.5–0.8 *cun* deep. Perform the reinforcing-reducing needle method with twirling. Reinforce deficiency and reduce excess. Leave the needles in place for 2–5 min. Insert the needles alternately into the points on each side. After treatment with this method for 1 week, the disease can be relieved.

Lobar Pneumonia

Dazhui (GV14)
Taodao (GV13)
Shenzhu (GV12)
Shendao (GV11)
Lingtai (GV10)
Zhiyang (GV9)
Jinsuo (GV8)
Zhongshu (GV7)
Jizhong (GV6)
Xuanshu (GV5)
Mingmen (GV4)
Yaoyangguan (GV3)
Yaoshu (GV2)
Changqiang (GV1)

Xiguan (LR7)
Yinlingquan (SP9)
6 cun
Zhongdu (LR6)
Lougu (SP7)
Ligou (LR5)
7 cun

Section Three

Diseases of the Digestive System

Stomach Ache

Treatment of stomach ache with acupuncture on paired points was first recorded by Huangfu Mi in his book Zhenjiu Jiayijing during the Jin Dynasty (266–420 A.D.). He wrote that stomach distension could be treated with acupuncture on the Zhongwan (CV12) and Zhangmen (LR13). He thought that diseases of the stomach should be treated with acupuncture on the front-mu points of the stomach and spleen meridians. During the Tang Dynasty (618–907 A.D.), Sun Simiao wrote in his book Qianjin Yaofang that the Geshu (BL17) and Yingu (KI10) can be used for treating bloating, stomach ache, ascites, and muscle aches. He also recorded that the Burong (ST19) and Qimen (LR14) could be used for treating stomach ache and acid reflux. He believed that points on the foot Shaoyin meridian and foot Jueyin meridian should be selected for treating stomach ache Wang Zhizhong in the Song Dynasty (960–1279 A.D.) recorded in his book Zhenjiu Zishengjing that the Xialian (LI8) and Xuanzhong (GB39) could be used for treating stomach heat and lack of appetite. The Xialian (LI8) is on the hand Yangming meridian, whereas the Xuanzhong (GB39) is on the foot Taiyang meridian. Zhao Ji in the Song Dynasty (960–1279 A.D.) wrote in his book Shengji Zonglu that stomach ache can be treated with acupuncture on the Dadu (SP2) and Taibai (SP3). Li Ting in the Ming Dynasty (1368–1644 A.D.) recorded in his book Yixue Rumen that abdominal pain can be treated with acupuncture on the Gongsun (SP4) and Neiguan (PC6).

Neiguan (PC6)–Zusanli (ST36)

Acupuncture is performed. Insert the needles perpendicularly into the Neiguan (PC6) on both sides at 0.5–1 *cun* deep. Next, insert the needles perpendicularly into the Zusanli (ST36) on both sides. Perform strong stimulation on all points. At the Neiguan (PC6), the patient will feel the needle pricking sensation radiating

upward to the armpits and downward to the middle fingers. At the Zusanli (ST36), the patient will feel the needle pricking sensation radiating to the back of the feet and feel heaviness in the legs. Leave the needles in place for 30 min. Perform this therapy daily.

Case: Ms. Zhao, a 50-year-old woman, suffered from chronic gastritis. She presented with persistent pain in the upper abdomen accompanied with nausea and vomiting.

Examination: She had a string-like slight rapid pulse and a red tongue with slightly yellow greasy fur. We treated her with this method. She was cured after three sessions of treatment.

Stomach Ache

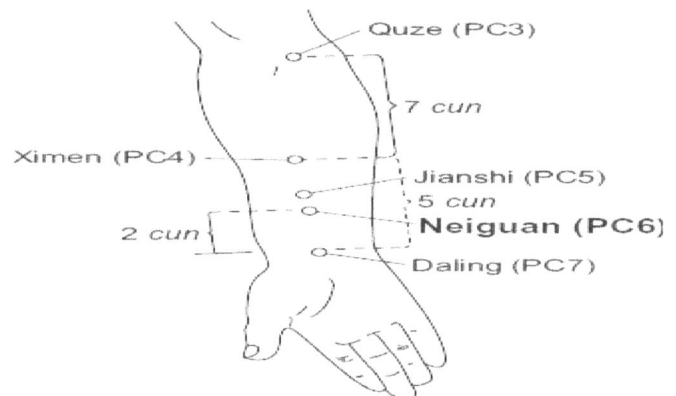

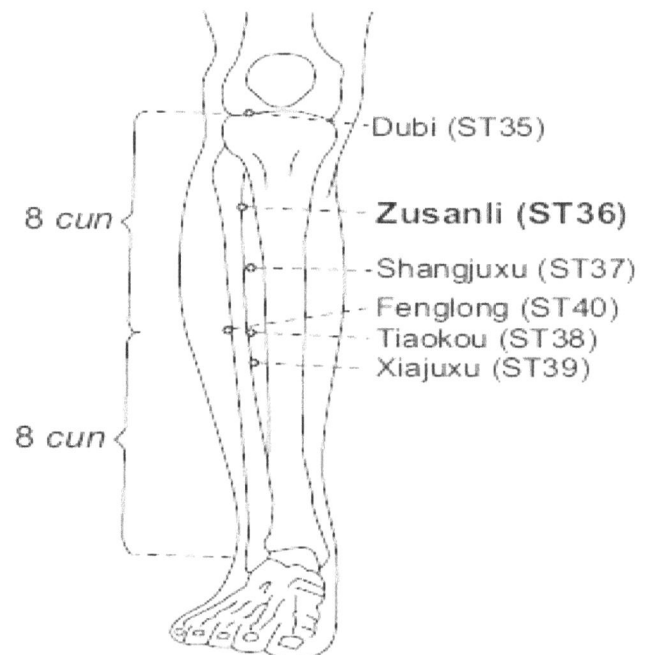

Stomach Ache

Stomach ache is often caused by transverse dysfunction of the Liver Wood offending the stomach or by spleen and stomach damaged by irregular diet and overwork. The Neiguan (PC6) is a Luo-connecting point of the hand Jueyin meridian. It connects to the triple energizers. Acupuncture on the Neiguan (PC6) can regulate Qi movement of the triple energizers. The Zusanli (ST36) is the He sea point of the foot Yangming meridian. Modern study has shown that acupuncture on the Zusanli (ST36) can contract the relaxed stomach, relax the contracted stomach, and relieve pyloric spasms. This pair of points can be used for invigorating the spleen, harmonizing the stomach, regulating Qi flow, and stopping pain.

Yintang–Liangqiu (ST34)–Tushui (22.11)

We have used these points as assistant points when treating acute stomach ache with the abovementioned pair of points. We achieved an unexpected effect, which was faster than taking pain relievers.

Case: Steve, a 21-year-old man, liked drinking cold beverages. Severe stomach ache developed in the patient approximately 30 min after playing basketball and drinking a cold beverage. When he came to our clinic, he was pressing his upper abdomen. He had a pale face, plump tongue with teeth-prints and white fur, and a weak pulse. He presented with abdominal rebound tenderness. Approximately 5 min after performing acupuncture, the pain disappeared completely. We performed moxibustion on the Zhongwan (CV12) once to cure the condition.

Stomach Ache

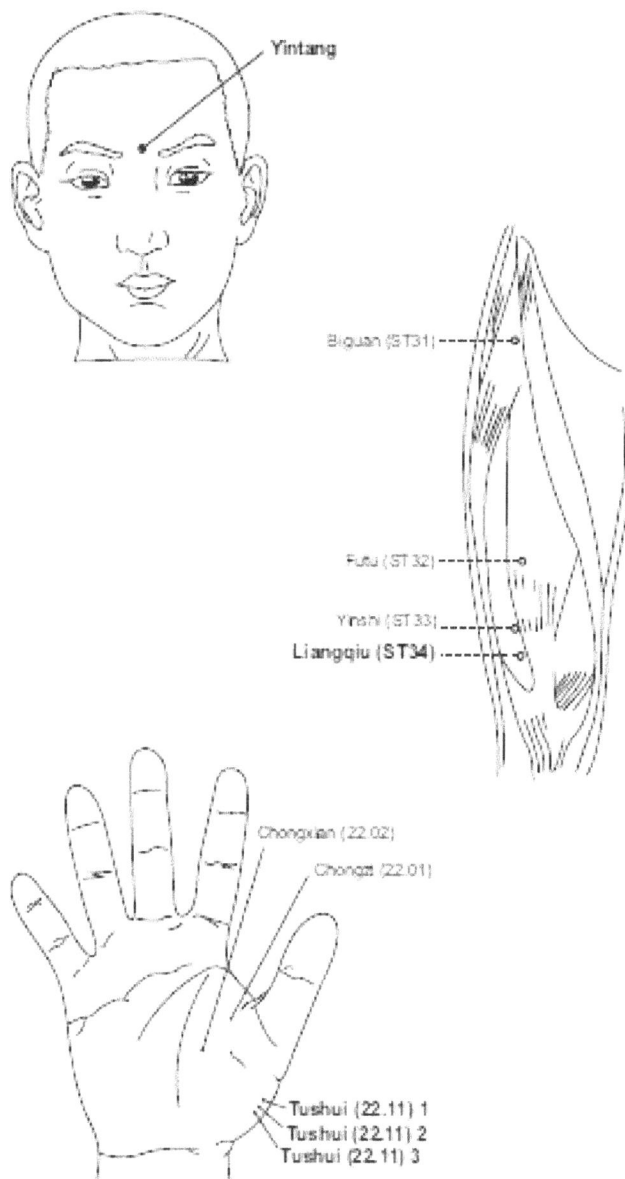

Regurgitation

Regurgitation

Formula One: Wei (Eye point)–Zhongjiao (Eye point)

Acupuncture is performed for 5 min. Leave the needles in place for 10 min. At the same time, perform moxibustion on the Zhong Kui. Normally, bloating, belching, and acid regurgitation due to overconsumption of greasy foods can be treated with this pair of points. The treatment is effective in a short time.

Formula Two: Hegu (LI4)–Zusanli (ST36)

Acupuncture is performed. Insert the needles perpendicularly at 1–1.2 *cun* deep, performing the reducing needle technique.

Case: Ms. Guo, a 13-year-old girl, suffered from stomach ache, lack of appetite, vomiting, and acid regurgitation. The pain started after eating and caused vomiting when it was severe. Treatment with western medicine did not improve the symptoms and the vomiting became worse. She became weak and tired. We treated her with this method, and after one session of treatment, she was cured.

Hegu (LI4)

Other name: Hukou

Yuan (Source) point

Location: On the dorsum of the hand, between the first and second metacarpal bones, in the middle of the second metacarpal bone on the radial side.

An easier way to locate: Put your thumb at the web of the first and second finger of another hand, with the distal crease of the thumb at the edge of the web. The Hegu (LI4) is under the tip of your thumb. (Figure 3–8)

Anatomy keys: Dorsal digital veins and the superficial branch of the radial nerve.

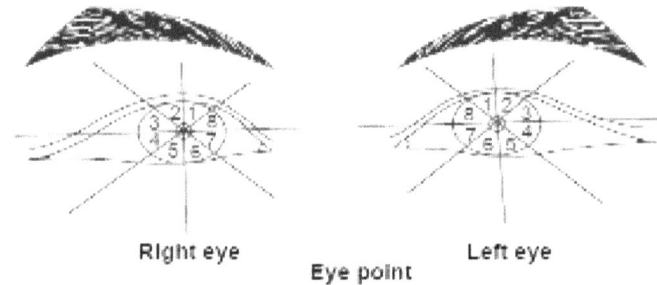

Right eye   Left eye
Eye point

1. Fei Dachang (Lung and large intestine)
2. Shen Pangguang (Kidney and bladder)
3. Shangjiao (Upper Energizer)
4. Gandan (Liver and gallbladder)
5. Zhongjiao (Middle Energizer)
6. Xin Xiaochang (Heart and small intestine)
7. Piwei (Spleen and stomach)
8. Xiajiao (Lower Energizer)

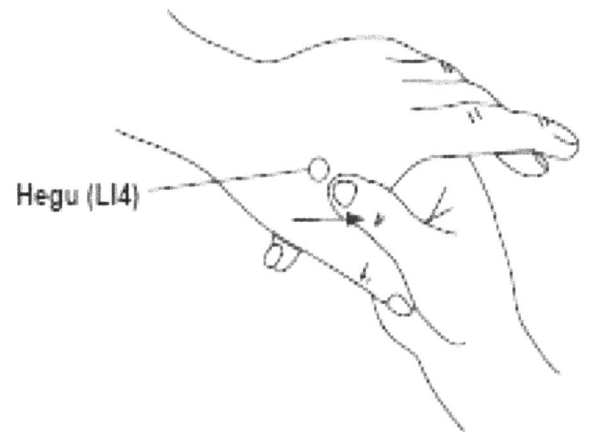

Hegu (LI4)

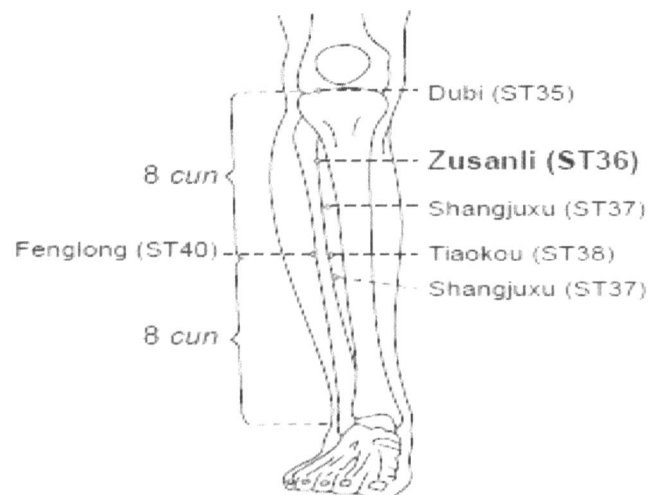

Dubi (ST35)
8 cun
Zusanli (ST36)
Shangjuxu (ST37)
Fenglong (ST40)
Tiaokou (ST38)
Shangjuxu (ST37)
8 cun

Hiccups

Hiccups

Neiguan (PC6)–Taichong (LR3)

Acupuncture is performed. Insert the needles perpendicularly into the Neiguan (PC6) and Taichong (LR3) on both sides at 0.5–1 cun deep. Perform strong stimulation on the Taichong (LR3). Leave the needles in place for 15–20 min.

We used this method for treating hiccups in two cases. One patient was cured after one session of treatment and the other was cured after two sessions of treatments.

Case: Mr. Huang, a 25-year-old man, suddenly developed hiccups after catching a cold 2 days earlier. He had a pale face, white watery tongue fur, and a slow pulse. The hiccup sounds were slow and powerful. He was cured after one session of treatment.

The hiccups in this case were caused by Qi stagnation and deficiency of liver and kidney. The liver controls conveyance and dispersion and regulates Qi movement. The liver meridian passes through two sides of the upper abdomen and diaphragm. The Taichong (LR3) is the Yuan source point of the liver meridian, which is the source of Qi. Acupuncture on the Taichong (LR3) can disperse liver, regulate Qi, and descend adverse Qi (when the disease develops in the upper body, select points in the lower body). The Neiguan (PC6) is the Luo-connect point of the hand Jueyin meridian. It connects to the Yinwei meridian and can be matched to the foot Yangming meridian. Acupuncture on the Neiguan (PC6) can descend adverse Qi in many meridians and regulate Qi movement of organs, thereby stopping hiccups.

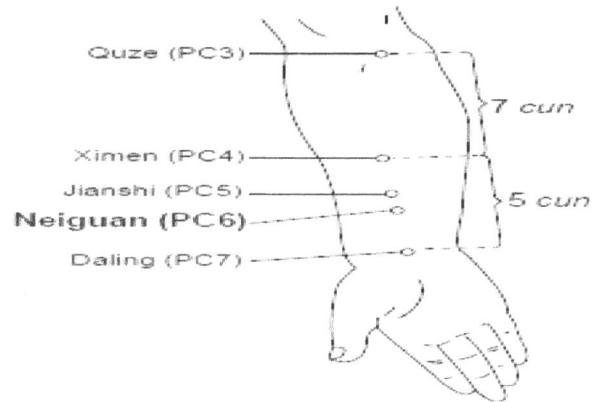

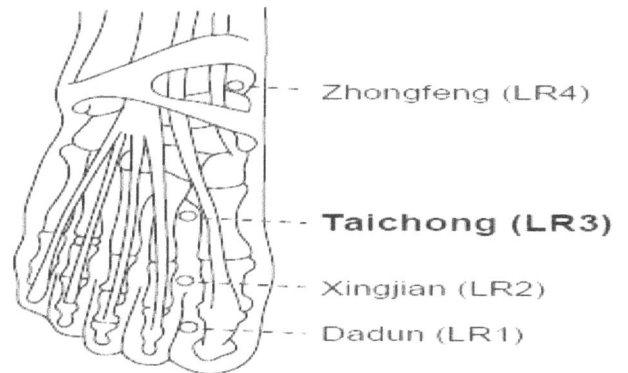

Gastroptosis

Gastroptosis

Tiwei–Shangfanying

Tiwei: Two extra points located at 4 *cun* lateral to the Zhongwan (CV12).

Shangfanying: An extra point located 1–3 finger breadths under the xiphoid process and 1–1.5 cm lateral of the midline of the abdomen.

Acupuncture is performed with the reducing needle technique and strong stimulation. Insert the needles approximately 1.5 *cun* deep. We used this method for treating gastoptosis in 60 cases. It was effective in relieving pain in all cases. Several points to be noted: 1. the patient should fast before acupuncture, 2. the patient should lie down and rest for 3 h after treatment and lie down frequently during the first 3 days after treatment, 3. the patient should eat frequent small meals that are easy to digest and full of nutrition, and 4. the patient can be slightly active after 10 days as long as the abdomen is not be strained. The patient should avoid heavy work for 2 months after treatment.

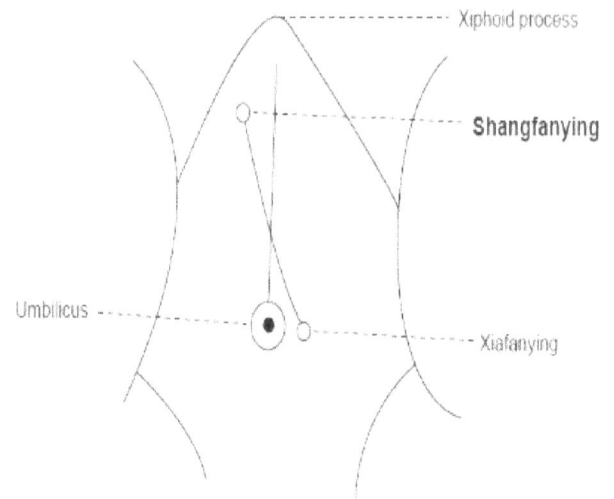

Gastric Neurosis

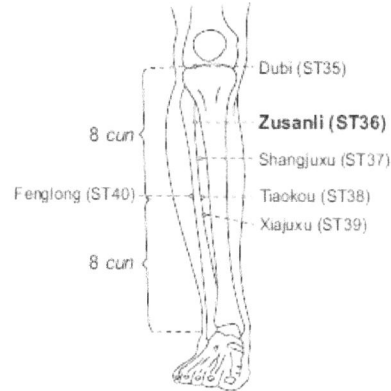

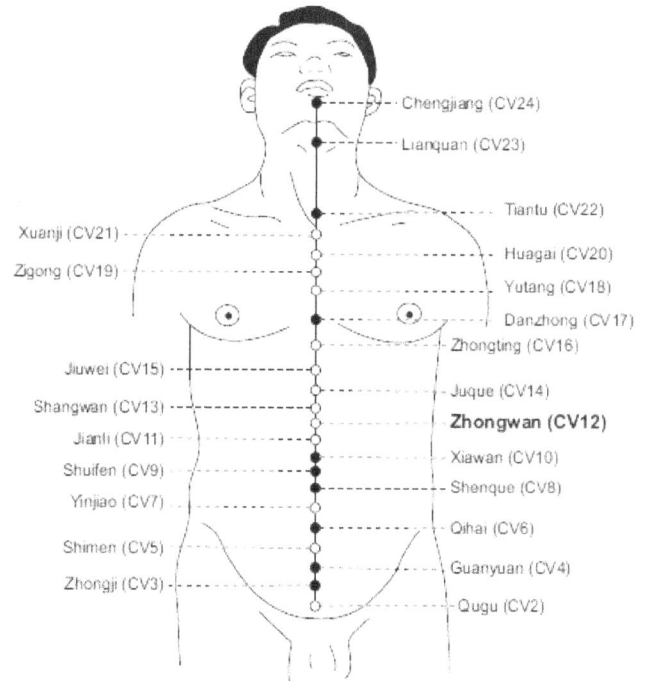

Zusanli (ST36)–Zhongwan (CV12)

Acupuncture is performed with strong stimulation. Insert the needles deeply at approximately 1.5–2 *cun*.

Case: Ms. Xiaochuan, a 27-year-old woman, reported an irritable mood. One year earlier, she developed insomnia, lack of appetite, nausea, vomiting, bloating after eating, and weakness in the extremities after quarreling with her neighbor. She was diagnosed with gastric neurosis. She took western medicine for 1 year, but there was no improvement. Belching, hiccups, and abdominal pain developed in the patient. She was introduced to our clinic by a friend. We treated her with this method. After two sessions of treatment and combining the treatment with the administration of the *Chaihu Shugan* decoction, she was cured.

Zusanli (ST36) is the He sea point of the stomach meridian. It can be used for regulating Qi movement of the middle energizer, harmonizing the stomach, and stopping pain as well as for regulating disorders of the autonomic nerves. The Zhongwan (CV12) is the front-mu point of the stomach and the convergence point of the viscera. It can be used for increasing movement of the stomach. This pair of points can be used for harmonizing the stomach, descending adverse Qi, and regulating nerve disorders.

Gastric Neurosis

Irritable Bowel Syndrome

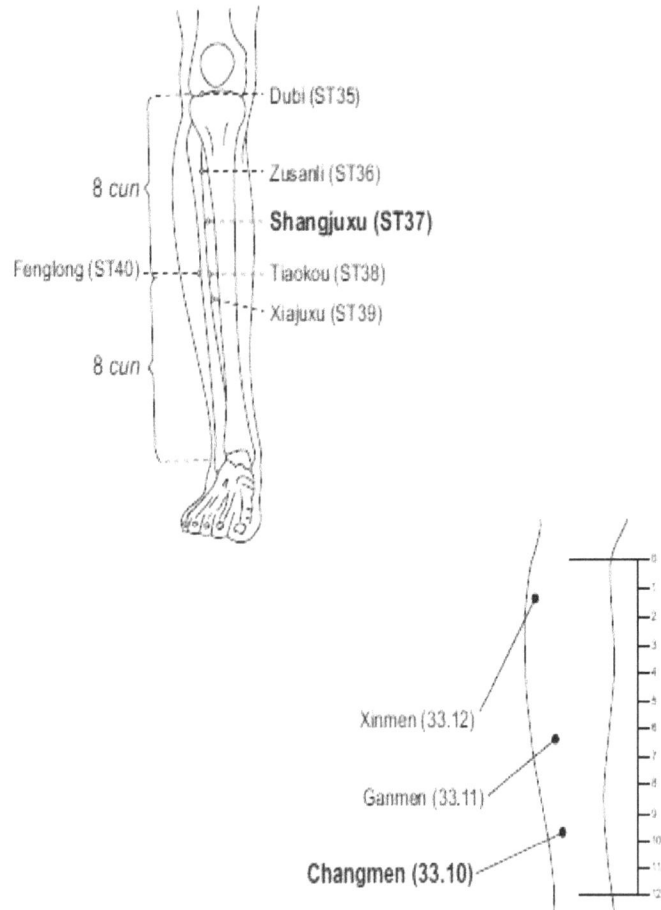

Changmen (33.10)–Shangjuxu (ST37)

Acupuncture is performed. Insert the needles perpendicularly at 1.5 *cun* deep.

Changmen (33.10): Located at the same place as the Zhizheng (SI7).

We have used this method for treating diseases of the intestine. In addition, this pair of points can be used for treating acute diarrhea and bacillary dysentery. This treatment is immediately effective.

Irritable Bowel Syndrome

Acute Gastroenteritis

Acute Gastroenteritis

Neiguan (PC6)–Taixi (KI3)

Acupuncture and warming needle moxibustion are performed. Insert the needles perpendicularly into the Neiguan (PC6) on both sides at 0.5–1 *cun* deep. Manipulate the needles occasionally. Leave the needles in place for 20 min. Perform warming needle moxibustion on the Taixi (KI3) with 10 Moxa cones.

Case: Mr. Chen, a 35-year-old waiter, developed abdominal pain, fever and diarrhea 5–6 times, and vomiting 2 times after eating seafood and drinking fruit juice. He was sent to the emergency room. At that time, he felt dizzy. His temperature was 37.8°C, blood pressure was 10.7/7 KPa, and pulse rate was 70 beats/min. His white blood cell counts were 10.8×10^9/L, with neutrophil counts at 0.9 and lymphocyte counts at 0.1. He was diagnosed with acute gastroenteritis and treated with fluid infusion, anti-shock medication, and anti-infection medication. However, his condition remained unstable. After 3 days, he developed diaphragmatic spasms. He was introduced to our clinic by his relatives. When he visited our clinic, he had a pale complexion, cold extremities, recurrent hiccups, and a faint and fine pulse. We treated him once with this method. After treatment, his blood pressure was 14.4–14.7/9.06–9.33 KPa and his heart rate was restored to 66–68 beats/min. After observation for 1 hour, the symptoms did not recur. The patient was subsequently discharged.

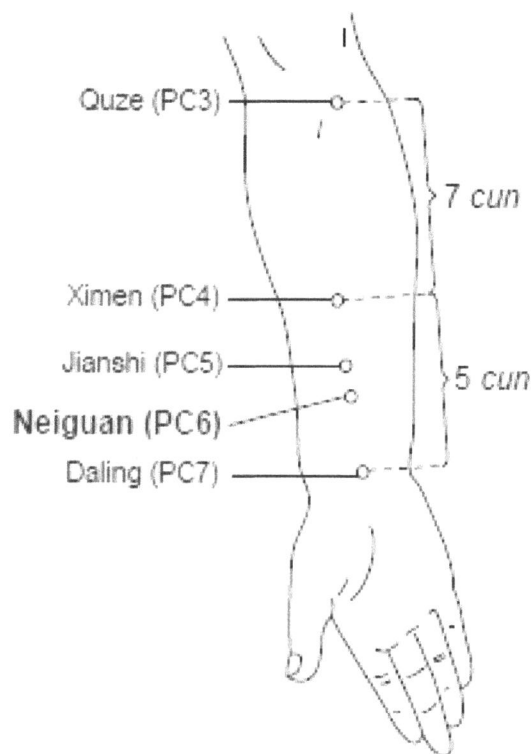

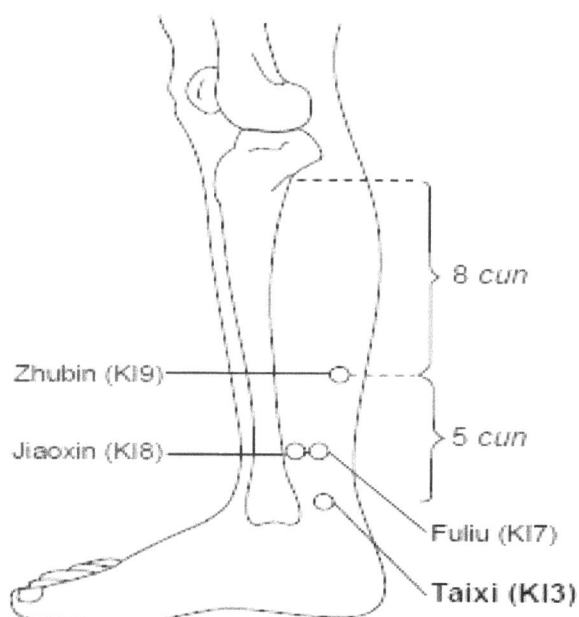

81

Diarrhea

Formula One: Dachang (Eye point)–Xiaochang (Eye point)

Acupuncture is performed. After achieving the needle pricking sensation, leave the needles in place for 15 min.

Formula Two: Pi (Hand point)–Yinbai (SP1)

Pi (Hand point): Located at the palmar aspect of the hand, i.e., at the midpoint of the finger crease on the thumb.

Acupuncture is performed using the uniform reinforcing–reducing needle technique. Leave the needles in place for 15 min or directly perform moxibustion.

Case: Mr. Li, a 38-year-old worker, developed watery diarrhea 1 day earlier after eating raw and cold food. He had trouble sleeping. He had abdominal pain and borborygmus, without burning pain in the anus or tenesmus. He self-medicated with antidiarrheal medications, but they were not effective. We treated him with this method once, and he was cured after the treatment.

Diarrhea

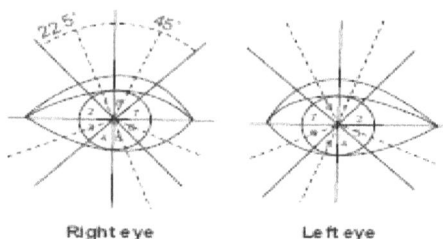

Right eye   Left eye

1. Shen Pangguang (kidney and bladder)
2. Shangjiao (Upper Energizer)
3. Gandan (liver and gallbladder)
4. Zhongjiao (Middle Energizer)
5. Xin Xiaochang (Heart and small intestine)
6. Piwei (Spleen and stomach)
7. Xiajiao (Lower Energizer)
8. Fei Dachang (Lung and large intestine)

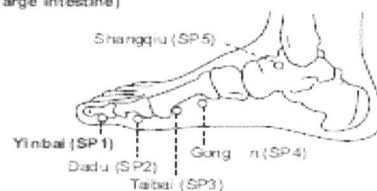

Shangqiu (SP5)
Yinbai (SP1)
Dadu (SP2)   Gongsun (SP4)
Taibai (SP3)

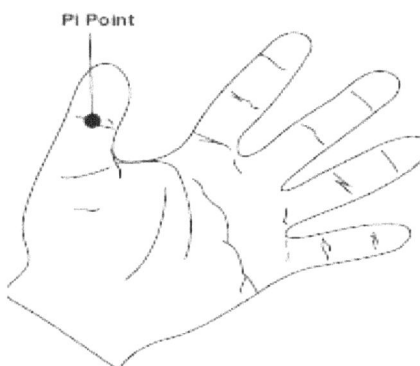

Pi Point

82

Gastric and Duodenal Ulcers

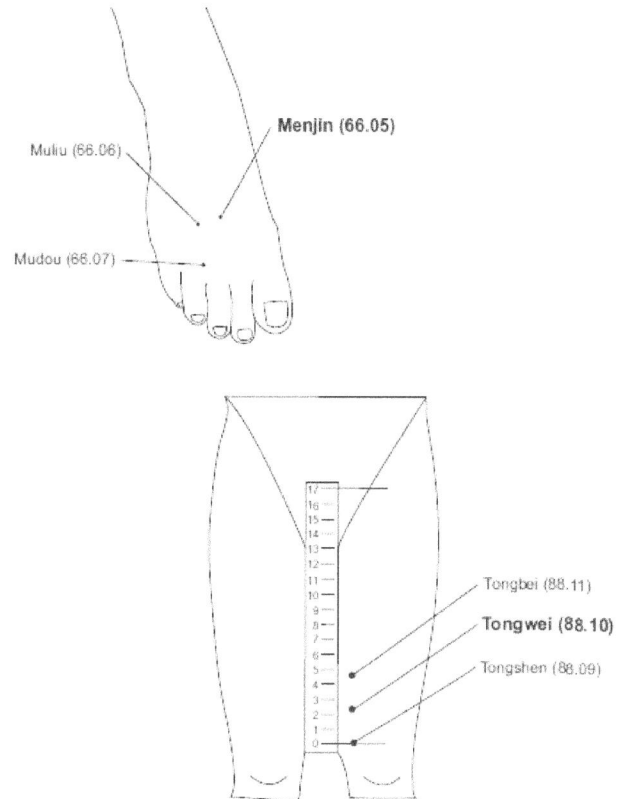

Gastric and Duodenal Ulcers

Menjin (66.05)–Tongwei (88.10)

Acupuncture is performed. To treat gastric and duodenal ulcers, we have tried many pairs of points. We found that this pair has the most stable effect. However, the effect depends on the practitioner's knowledge about the Dong needle technique. Even though many authors of books on the Dong needle technique know the points, they know less about the anatomy and application of the technique. It is dangerous for common practitioners to perform acupuncture if they have little knowledge about the points and anatomy. We advise practitioners to not perform acupuncture on patients thoughtlessly. Otherwise, the consequences may be disastrous.

Constipation

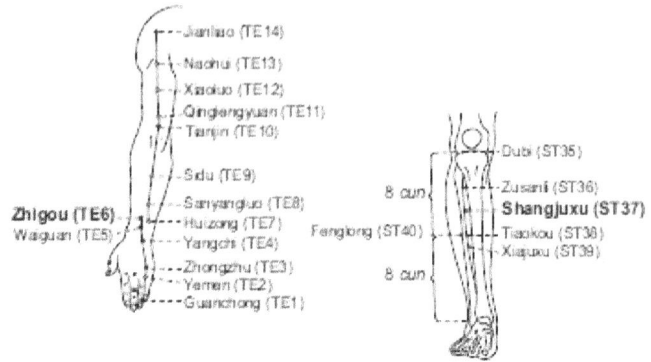

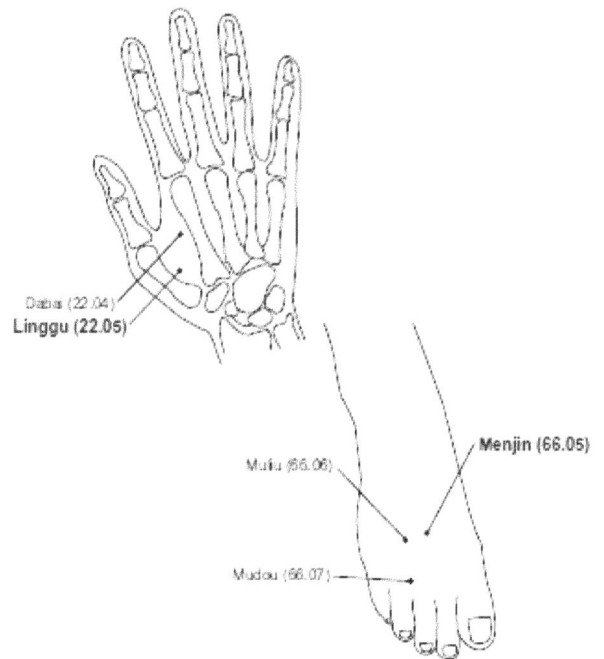

Formula One: Zhigou (TE6)–Shangjuxu (ST37)

Acupuncture is performed. Insert the needles perpendicularly into the Zhigou (TE6) on both sides at 0.8–1.2 *cun* deep. Insert the needles perpendicularly into the Shangjuxu (ST37) on both sides at 1–2 *cun* deep, performing the reducing needle technique.

Case: Mr. Li, a 30-year-old stevedore, suffered from constipation for many years. He was treated by an enema at a western medicine clinic. The symptom improved for approximately 6 months, but did not disappear completely. When he visited our clinic, he had a dry mouth, irritable mood, bloating, troubles with bowel movement, infrequent urination, yellow greasy tongue fur, and a string-like rapid pulse. After two sessions of treatment with this method, constipation did not recur.

Formula Two: Linggu (22.05)–Menjin (66.05)

We performed the needle control technique on this pair of points for treating severe constipation. After two sessions of treatment, the condition was cured. This is presented for reference.

Abdominal Distension

Treatment of abdominal distension with acupuncture on paired points was first recorded by Huangfu Mi in his book Zhenjiu Jiayijing during the Jin Dynasty (266–420 A.D.). He said that abdominal distension, which can cause back pain and increased appetite without weight gain, can be treated by acupuncture on the Pishu (BL20) and Jixie. Jixie is another name for Zhangmen (LR13).

Zusanli (ST36)–Menjin (66.05)

Acupuncture is performed. The key is to find the correct location of the points and to not insert the needles too deeply. Usually, the needles are inserted at approximately 5–8 *fen*. Ask the patient to breathe in deeply. Often, the patient will soon pass gas and feel comfortable. During treatment, spicy and pungent foods and cold drinks should be avoided.

Case: Ms. Wang, a 27-year-old woman, was often on a diet. She had gastritis for many years and poor function of the intestines. She usually belched, felt bloated, and had trouble passing gas. After treatment with this method, she passed gas and felt comfortable. The treatment was immediately effective. This is presented for reference.

Abdominal Distension

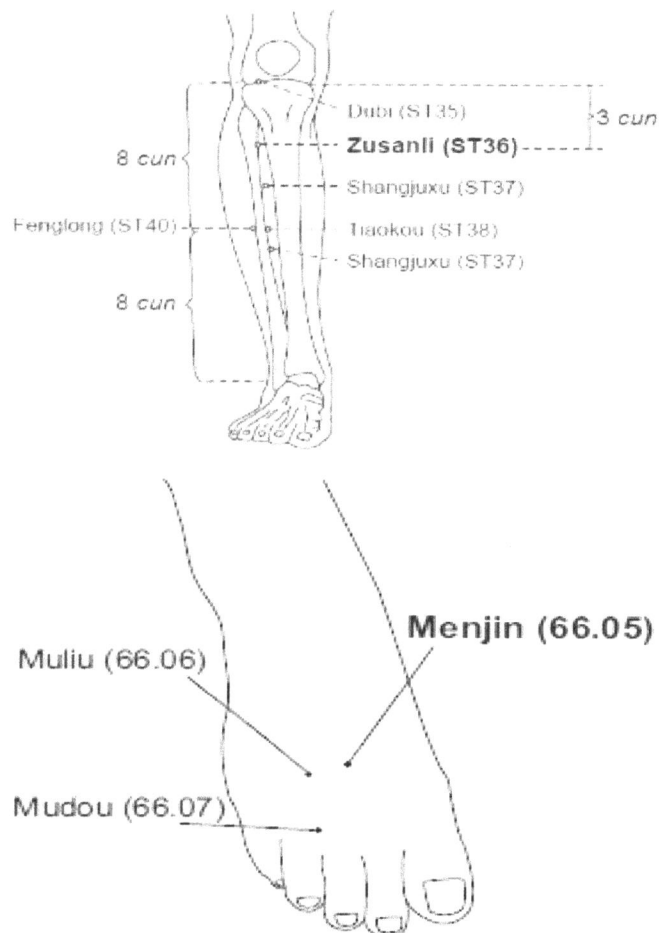

Liver Cancer

Liver Cancer

This disease does not develop in a short period. Thus, it is desirable to know more about patients with this disease. Most of them have a history of hepatitis. The prevalence rate of hepatitis is very high in mainland China, southeastern Asia, and Taiwan.

Ganyan–Zusanli (ST36)

Ganyan: An extra point located 2 *cun* beneath the lower edge of the costal arch on the right midclavicular line.

Acupuncture is performed. Insert a needle perpendicularly into Ganyan at 0.5–1 *cun* deep. Slowly insert the needles perpendicularly into the Zusanli (ST36) on both sides. Do not lift or thrust the needles. Leave the needles in place for 15–30 min.

Case: Mr. Wang, a 45-year-old man, was diagnosed with liver cancer. We performed acupuncture, and the effect was satisfactory. We combined herbal medicine with acupuncture. His pain was relieved after treatment.

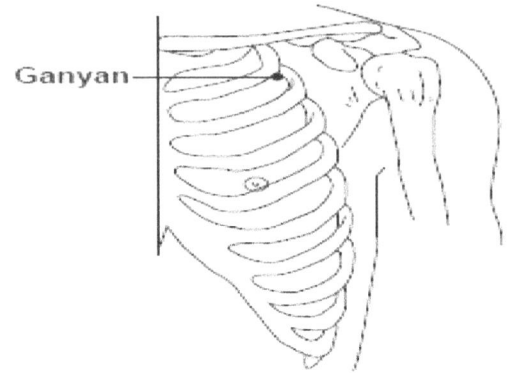

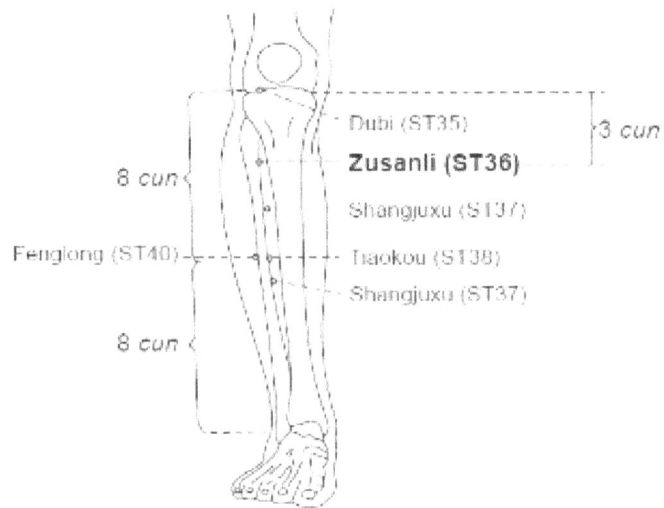

Chapter Five

Diseases of the Urogenital System

Impotence

There are few records in ancient books about the treatment of impotence with acupuncture on paired points. Li Xuechuan in the Qing Dynasty (1636–1912 A.D.) recorded in his book Zhenjiu Fengyuan that impotence and deficient cold of the kidney and bladder can be cured by moxibustion on the Shenshu (BL23) and Qihai (CV6).

Formula One: Huiyin (CV1)–Guanyuan (CV4)

Acupuncture is performed with the patient in the lithotomy position. Insert a needle perpendicularly into the Huiyin (CV1) at 2–3 *cun* deep. Twist and twirl the needle slightly, making the needle pricking sensation radiate to the tip of the penis. Vibrate the needle slightly for 1–3 min and then remove the needle. Insert another needle into the Guanyuan (CV4) perpendicularly or obliquely toward the pubic symphysis at 2–2.5 *cun* deep. After achieving the needle pricking sensation, manipulate the needle so that the needle pricking sensation radiates to the perineal region. Continue twisting and twirling for 3–5 min before removing the needle.

Formula Two: Huoying (66.03)–Qiyang

Qiyang is a secret point of Tong. It is shared here for reference. It is located at the midpoint of the lower edge of the pubic symphysis.

Acupuncture is performed, without any specific needle technique. Leave the needles in place for 30 min. Perform moxibustion at the same time.

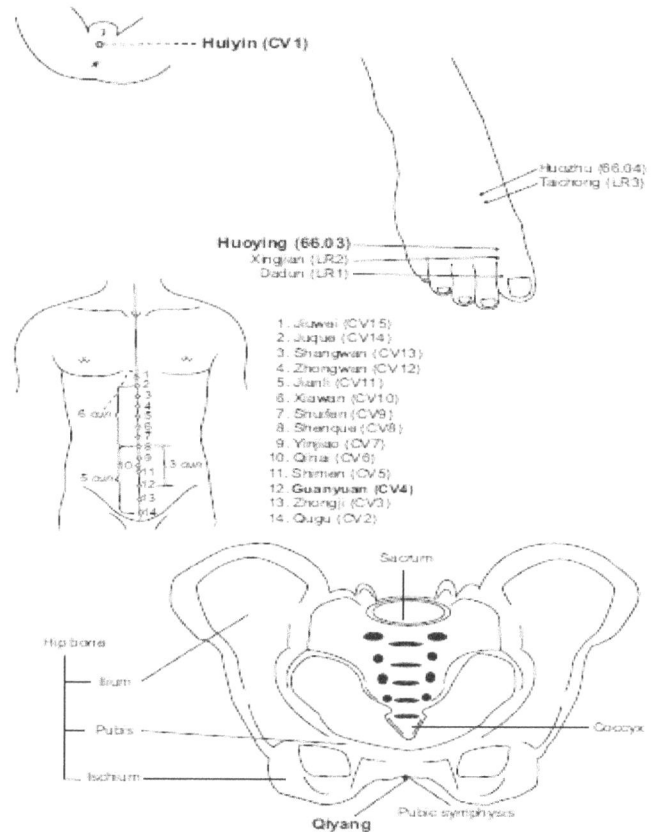

Spermatorrhea

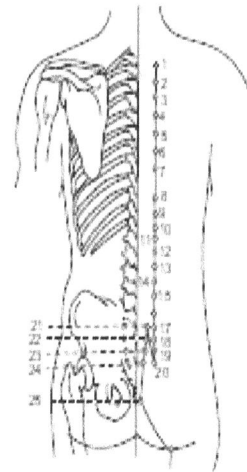

Spermatorrhea is a sexual disorder caused by dysfunction of the cerebral cortex and central nerve. When sexual excitation is enhanced, the patient may suffer from emission of semen without intercourse.

Formula One: Huiyin (CV1)–Baliao [including Shangliao (BL31), Ciliao (BL32), Zhongliao (BL33), and Xialiao (BL34)]

Acupuncture is performed. Insert the needles perpendicularly into the points approximately 1–1.5 *cun* deep, without any specific needle technique.

Formula Two: Xiasanhuang (77.17, 77.19, 77.21)– Yingu (KI10)

Insert the needles obliquely into the Xiasanhuang (77.17, 77.19, 77.21) approximately 2–2.5 *cun* deep. Ask the patient to lie down. Insert the needles perpendicularly into the Yingu (KI10) approximately 1.5 *cun* deep, performing the reinforcing needle technique.

Spermatorrhea

1. Dazhu (BL11)
2. Fengmen (BL12)
3. Feishu (BL13)
4. Jueyinshu (BL14)
5. Xinshu (BL15)
6. Dushu (BL16)
7. Geshu (BL17)
8. Ganshu (BL18)
9. Danshu (BL19)
10. Pishu (BL20)
11. Weishu (BL21)
12. Sanjiaoshu (BL22)
13. Shenshu (BL23)
14. Qihaishu (BL24)
15. Dachangshu (BL25)
16. Guanyuanshu (BL26)
17. Xiaochangshu (BL27)
18. Pangguangshu (BL28)
19. Zhonglvshu (BL29)
20. Baihuanshu (BL30)
21. **Shangliao (BL31)**
22. **Ciliao (BL32)**
23. **Zhongliao (BL33)**
24. **Xialiao (BL34)**
25. Huiyang (BL35)

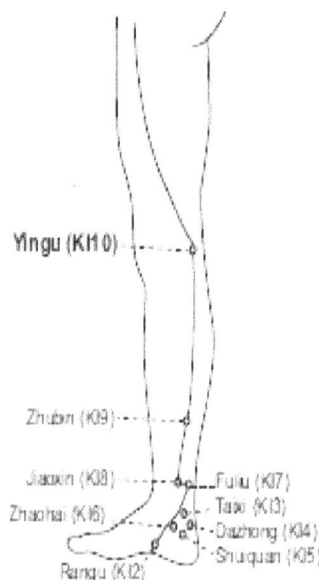

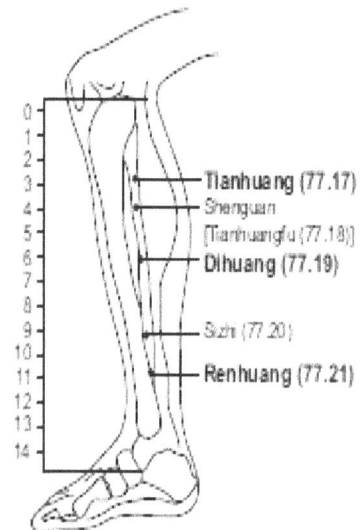

Yingu (KI10)

Zhubin (KI9)

Jiaoxin (KI8)
Zhaohai (KI6)
Rangu (KI2)

Fuliu (KI7)
Taixi (KI3)
Dazhong (KI4)
Shuiquan (KI5)

Tianhuang (77.17)
Shenguan [Tianhuangfu (77.18)]
Dihuang (77.19)
Sizhi (77.20)
Renhuang (77.21)

Infertility

Infertility

Taichong (LR3)–Dahe (KI12)

Acupuncture is performed. Insert a 2-*cun*-long filiform needle into the Taichong (LR3) approximately 1–1.5 *cun* deep, penetrating through the Yongquan (KI1). After lifting and thrusting the needle, leave the needle in place for 20 min. Then, insert another needle into the Dahe (KI12) while performing the same technique.

Case: Mr. Liu, a 29-year-old man, had been married for 6 years but could not have a baby. He had trouble ejaculating during intercourse. He had a pink tongue with little fur and a string-like thready pulse. After two sessions of treatment with this method, ejaculation became normal. After 2 months, he informed us that his wife was pregnant.

This disease is usually caused by liver depression transforming into fire. The fire offends the kidney, causing trouble with ejaculation. This method emphasizes on inserting the needle into the Taichong (LR3) while penetrating through the Yongquan (KI1) to reduce Liver Fire. Inserting the needle into the Dahe (KI12) is meant to reinforce the kidney and resume ejaculation.

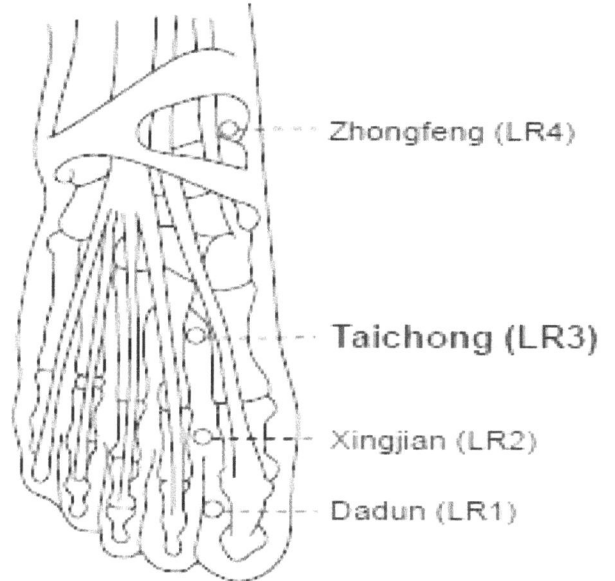

Zhongfeng (LR4)

Taichong (LR3)

Xingjian (LR2)

Dadun (LR1)

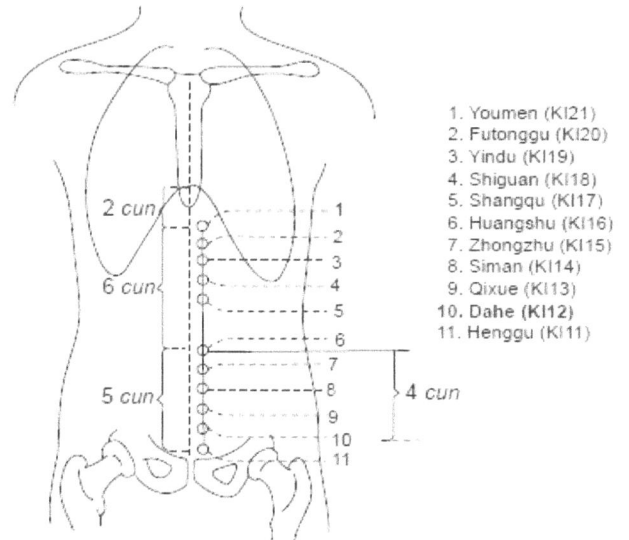

1. Youmen (KI21)
2. Futonggu (KI20)
3. Yindu (KI19)
4. Shiguan (KI18)
5. Shangqu (KI17)
6. Huangshu (KI16)
7. Zhongzhu (KI15)
8. Siman (KI14)
9. Qixue (KI13)
10. Dahe (KI12)
11. Henggu (KI11)

89

Erectile Dysfunction

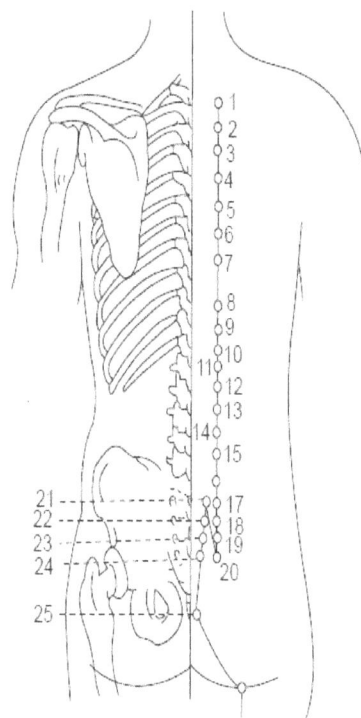

Erectile Dysfunction

Zhonglvshu (BL29)–Huiyang (BL35)

Acupuncture is performed. Slowly insert a 5-*cun*-long filiform needle into the Zhonglvshu (BL29), making the needle and skin form a 70° angle. When the needle penetrates the gluteus maximus, the practitioner should feel that the muscle is tightly pinched by the needle. Keep twisting and twirling the needle during insertion, radiating the needle pricking sensation to the perineal region. Insert another needle into the Huiyang (BL35) toward the pubic symphysis, radiating the needle pricking sensation to the perineal region. Manipulate the needles. Leave the needles in place for 20 min.

Case: Super, a 35-year-old fisherman, complained of problems with sexual activity for 1 year and six months. The problem was caused by nervousness on his wedding night. He took Viagra and felt better for approximately 1 week. Afterward, no treatment was effective. A friend suggested that he try alternative medicine. He usually suffered from palpitations, sweating, and weakness of the lower back and legs. He was slightly overweight and bald. He had a pale complexion, a plump and tender tongue with little fur, and a deep and fine pulse. After 6–7 treatments with this method, his penis could achieve erection in the morning. After one session of treatment, he could resume sexual activity. However, he still had some fears. After undergoing some sex education, he now lives a happy life with his wife.

1. Dazhu (BL11)
2. Fengmen (BL12)
3. Feishu (BL13)
4. Jueyinshu (BL14)
5. Xinshu (BL15)
6. Dushu (BL16)
7. Geshu (BL17)
8. Ganshu (BL18)
9. Danshu (BL19)
10. Pishu (BL20)
11. Weishu (BL21)
12. Sanjiaoshu (BL22)
13. Shenshu (BL23)
14. Qihaishu (BL24)
15. Dachangshu (BL25)
16. Guanyuanshu (BL26)
17. Xiaochangshu (BL27)
18. Pangguangshu (BL28)
19. **Zhonglvshu (BL29)**
20. Baihuanshu (BL30)
21. Shangliao (BL31)
22. Ciliao (BL32)
23. Zhongliao (BL33)
24. Xialiao (BL34)
25. **Huiyang (BL35)**

Koro (Retraction of Penis)

Koro (Retraction of Penis)

Hegu (LI4)–Taichong (LR3)

Electro-acupuncture is performed. Insert the needles perpendicularly into the Hegu (LI4) and Taichong (LR3) at 0.5 *cun* deep with strong stimulation. After achieving the needle pricking sensation, connect the needle handle to the electrode and supply power. Leave the needles in place for 20 min.

Koro (retraction of penis) is usually caused by excessive sexual activity, which can consume and impair the kidney essence. Pathogens can enter and offend the Shaoyin and Jueyin channels, which pass through the perineal region. As the saying goes, "impairment of the foot Jueyin, caused by internal pathogens, can cause impotence, and this impairment causes koro if it is caused by cold pathogens."

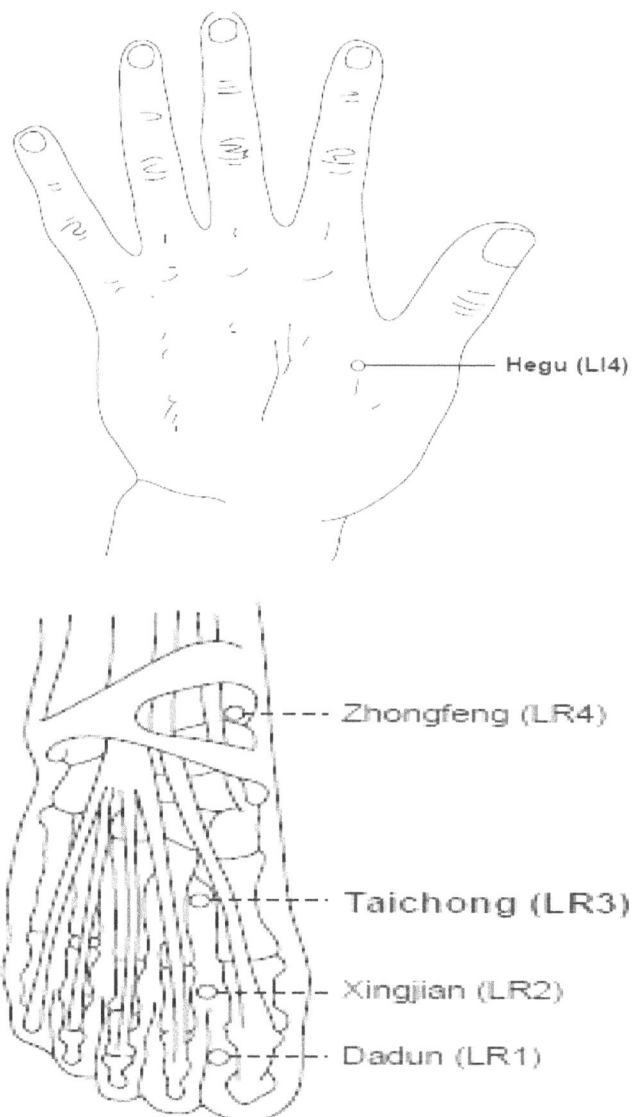

Hegu (LI4)

Zhongfeng (LR4)

Taichong (LR3)

Xingjian (LR2)

Dadun (LR1)

Dribbling and Retention of Urine

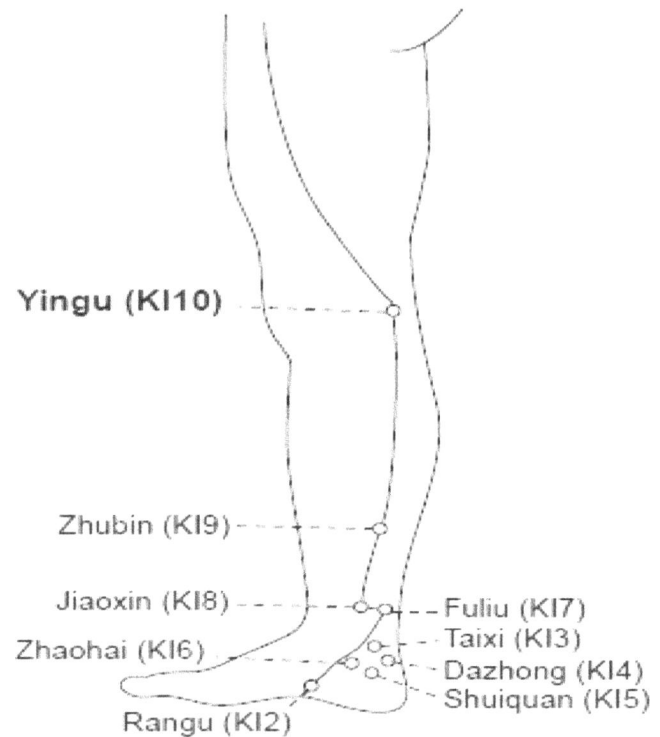

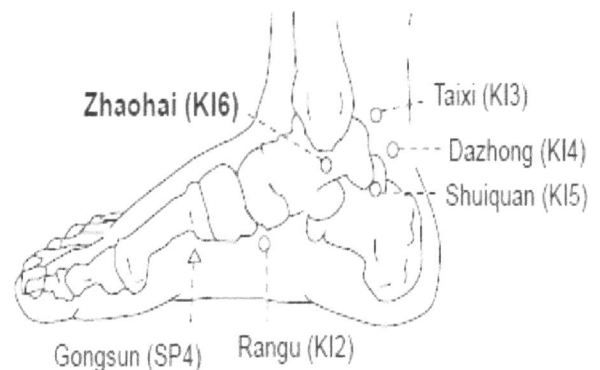

Dribbling and Retention of Urine

Yingu (KI10)–Zhaohai (KI6)

Acupuncture is performed. Insert 1.5-*cun*-long filiform needles perpendicularly into the Yingu (KI10) and Zhaohai (KI6) with strong stimulation. Leave the needles in place for 15 min.

Case: Mr. He, a 40-year-old worker, suffered from lumbar disc herniation and was treated with traction reduction. One week after therapy, he felt distention of the lower abdomen and had difficulty in urinating. He underwent catheterization and was administered medicines, but they were not effective. He was short of breath, unwilling to speak, and lacked an appetite. He had dry stool and a heavy sensation in his lower abdomen. He had pale tongue with thin fur and a deep, slow pulse. After treatment with this method, he felt the urge to urinate. After 1 hour, he could urinate freely.

Urine Retention

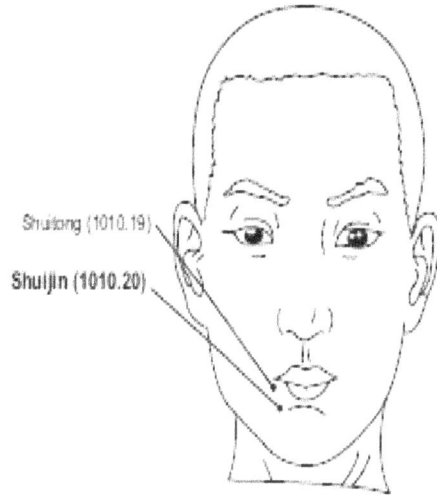

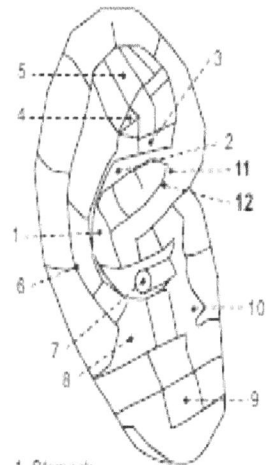

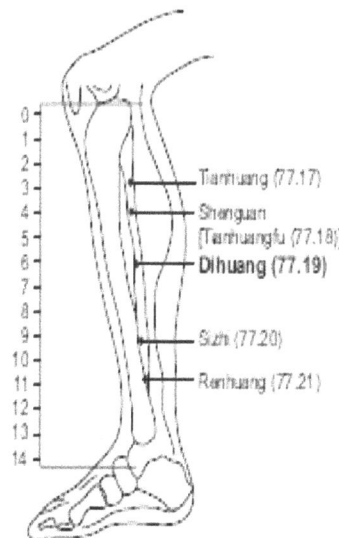

Formula One: Niaodao (Ear point)–Zhichang Xiaduan (Ear point)

Niaodao (Ear point): Located at the helix near the Pangguang (bladder) point.

Zhichang Xiaduan (Ear point): Located at the helix near the Dachang (large intestine) point.

Acupuncture is performed. Insert the needles into the Niaodao and Zhichang Xiaduan on both sides. After twisting and twirling, leave the needles in place for 5 min.

Case: Jiang underwent hemorrhoidectomy 10 years ago. Postoperatively, he had difficulty in urinating and felt distention of the lower abdomen and anus. After applying heat and body acupuncture, the symptoms were not relieved. He underwent catheterization twice, but could not urinate on his own. We treated him with this method. After 5 min, he could urinate on his own, which he described as miraculous.

Formula Two: Dihuang (77.19)–Shuijin (1010.20)

Dihuang (77.19): Insert the needles upward obliquely at a 45° angle, without any specific needle technique.

Shuijin (1010.20): Insert the needles inward, approximately 3 *fen* deep.

We have used Tong's needle technique for treating this disease. The effectiveness was immediate. This is provided as a reference.

Urine Retention

Shuitong (1010.19)
Shuijin (1010.20)

Tianhuang (77.17)
Shenguan [Tianhuangfu (77.18)]
Dihuang (77.19)
Sizhi (77.20)
Renhuang (77.21)

1. Stomach
2. Kidney
3. Sciatic nerve
4. Shenmen
5. Knee
6. Shoulder
7. Heart
8. Occiput
9. Eye
10. Endocrine
11. Niaodao
12. Zhichang Xiaduan

Urinary Incontinence

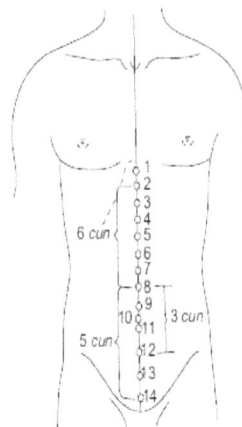

Urinary Incontinence

Urinary incontinence can be divided into two categories: true and pseudo. True urinary incontinence is caused by dysfunction of the bladder and sphincter. In pseudo urinary incontinence, the function of the sphincter is normal and it is caused by an overfull bladder. Urine strongly stimulates the wall of the bladder, causing the sphincter to relax.

In practice, there are more pseudo urinary incontinence cases than true urinary incontinence cases. In the theory of traditional Chinese medicine, this disease comprises enuresis.

Formula One: Leg motor and sensory area (Scalp acupuncture)–Sanyinjiao (SP6)

Acupuncture is performed with strong stimulation. Insert the needles at 1–1.5 *cun* deep, performing the uniform reinforcing–reducing needle technique. The needle pricking sensation will radiate forward to the perineal region. Leave the needles in place for 20 min. Next, perform moxibustion on these points with 5–7 moxa-cones.

Formula Two: Guanyuan (CV4)–Taixi (KI3)

Acupuncture is performed. Insert the needles perpendicularly into the Guanyuan (CV4) at 1.5–2 *cun* deep. Perform heat-producing needle technique, radiating the warm sensation to the perineal region. Next, insert the needles perpendicularly into the Taixi (KI3) at 0.5–1 *cun* deep, radiating the needle pricking sensation upward. Leave the needles in place for 20 min.

We have used this method for treating one case of urinary incontinence. The disease was cured after two treatments.

1. Jiuwei (CV15)
2. Juque (CV14)
3. Shangwan (CV13)
4. Zhongwan (CV12)
5. Jianli (CV11)
6. Xiawan (CV10)
7. Shuifen (CV9)
8. Shenque (CV8)
9. Yinjiao (CV7)
10. Qihai (CV6)
11. Shimen (CV5)
12. Guanyuan (CV4)
13. Zhongji (CV3)
14. Qugu (CV2)

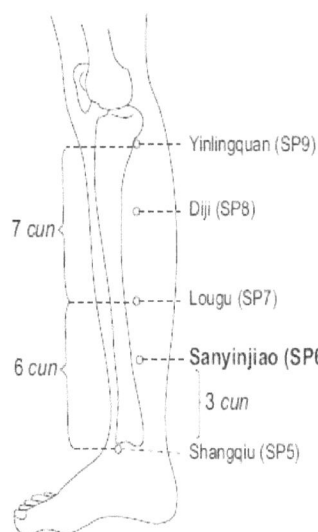

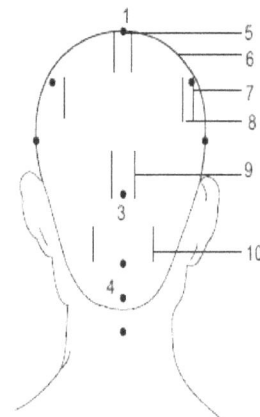

Yinlingquan (SP9)
Diji (SP8)
Lougu (SP7)
Sanyinjiao (SP6)
Shangqiu (SP5)

1. Midline of head
2. Parietal bone tuberde
3. External occipital protuberance
4. Back hairline
5. Leg motor and sensory area
6. Sensory area
7. Motor area
8. Speech #2 area
9. Vision area
10. Balance area

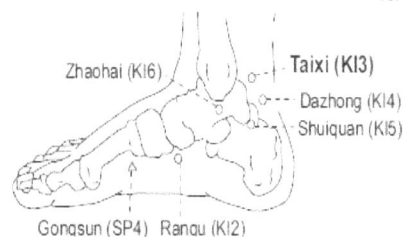

Zhaohai (KI6)
Taixi (KI3)
Dazhong (KI4)
Shuiquan (KI5)
Gongsun (SP4) Rangu (KI2)

Urination Dysfunction

Formula One: Tongshen (88.09)–Shangsanhuang (88.12, 88.13, 88.14)

Acupuncture is performed. Insert the needles 1 *cun* deep, without any specific needle technique.

We have used this pair of points for treating diseases of the urinary system.

Formula Two: Huiyang (BL35)–Xiasanhuang (77.17, 77.19, 77.21)

Acupuncture is performed. In practice, the Huiyang (BL35) can be used for treating many diseases, depending on the needle direction. For urine detention, the tip of the needle should be 100 mm deep toward the sacrum. The needle pricking sensation should radiate to the lower abdomen. For urinary incontinence, the tip of the needle should be 100 mm deep toward the urethra. The needle pricking sensation should radiate to the perineal region. Leave the needles in place for 20 min.

Urination Dysfunction

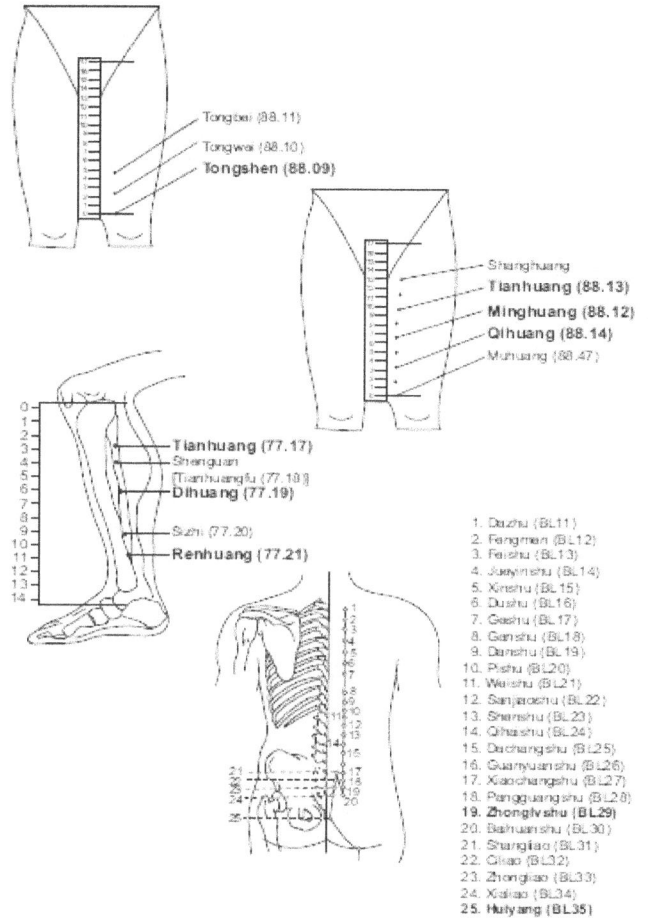

Tongbai (88.11)
Tongwei (88.10)
Tongshen (88.09)

Shanghuang
Tianhuang (88.13)
Minghuang (88.12)
Qihuang (88.14)
Muhuang (88.47)

Tianhuang (77.17)
Shenguan
[Tianhuangfu (77.18)]
Dihuang (77.19)

Suzhi (77.20)
Renhuang (77.21)

1. Dazhu (BL11)
2. Fengmen (BL12)
3. Feishu (BL13)
4. Jueyinshu (BL14)
5. Xinshu (BL15)
6. Dushu (BL16)
7. Geshu (BL17)
8. Ganshu (BL18)
9. Danshu (BL19)
10. Pishu (BL20)
11. Weishu (BL21)
12. Sanjiaoshu (BL22)
13. Shenshu (BL23)
14. Qihaishu (BL24)
15. Dachangshu (BL25)
16. Guanyuanshu (BL26)
17. Xiaochangshu (BL27)
18. Pangguangshu (BL28)
19. Zhonglvshu (BL29)
20. Baihuanshu (BL30)
21. Shangliao (BL31)
22. Ciliao (BL32)
23. Zhongliao (BL33)
24. Xialiao (BL34)
25. Huiyang (BL35)

Stranguria

Stranguria

The treatment of stranguria has been recorded by many ancient practitioners, with Sun Simiao in the Tang Dynasty (618–907 A.D.) being the first to record this in his book Qianjin Yaofang. He said that the Jingmen (GB25) and Zhaohai (KI6) could be used for treating yellow urine and difficulty in urination: "The Changqiang (GV1) and Xiaochangshu (BL27) can be used for treating difficulty in urination and bowel movement, stranguria, and dribbling of urine. Moxibustion can be performed on the point at 1.5 *cun* near the Xiayuquan (i.e., Zigong, EX-CA1) using 30 moxa-cones. Fill the navel with salt and perform moxibustion on it with moxa-cones."

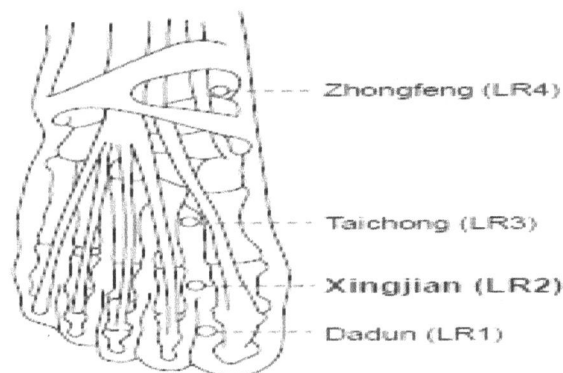

Xingjian (LR2)–Qugu (CV2)

Acupuncture is performed. Insert the needles into the Xingjian (LR2) on both sides and into the Qugu (CV2), performing the reducing needle technique. After achieving the needle pricking sensation, leave the needles in place for 20 min.

Case: Ms. Hua, a 20-year-old dealer, suffered from frequent urination for 3 days. Her urine was yellow and she experienced a burning sensation after urination. Treatment with western medicine was ineffective. She had the urge to urinate frequently. She had spasms in the lower abdomen, normal appetite, dry mouth, a bitter taste in her mouth, and a craving for cold drink and food. After two treatments with this method, the symptoms disappeared.

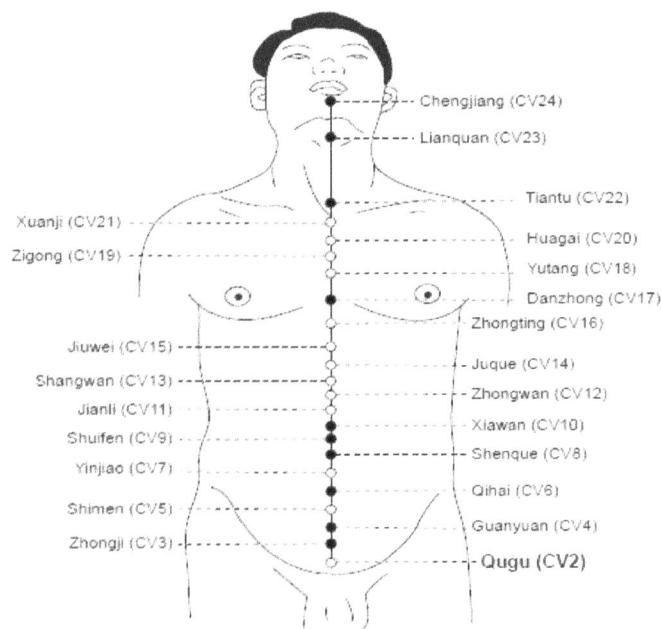

The liver meridian passes through the perineal region and urinary system. Therefore, Liver Fire can cause this disease. It should be treated by clearing the Liver Fire. Select the Xing-Spring point of the liver meridian, i.e., the Xinagjian (LR2) and Qugu (CV2), which is near the affected area, to clear the Liver Fire, according to the theory of the mother-son relationship.

Urinary System Infection

Urinary System Infection

Formula One: Shen (Eye point)–Xiajiao (Eye point)

Shen: Located on the second area around the eye.

Xiajiao: Located on the eighth area around the eye.

Acupuncture is performed. Insert needles measuring (0.27–0.32) * 15 mm into the areas. After achieving the needle pricking sensation, leave the needles in place for 20–30 min.

Formula Two: Sanyinjiao (SP6)–Zhongfeng (LR4)

Acupuncture is performed. Insert the needles obliquely into the Sanyinjiao (SP6) at 1.5 *cun* deep, performing the reducing needle technique. Insert the needles perpendicularly into the Zhongfeng (LR4) at 1.5 *cun* deep with strong stimulation. Leave the needles in place for 20 min.

What are the main factors for efficacy of acupuncture? First, efficacy depends on proper syndrome differentiation, without which it is impossible to select the proper points. When treating diseases, the location (viscera and channels) of the diseases should be known. Syndrome differentiation includes comprehensive analysis of information gained using the four diagnostic methods (i.e., observing, smelling and listening, inquiring, and diagnosing via palpation and pulse), Dong's palm diagnosis, and syndrome differentiation theory.

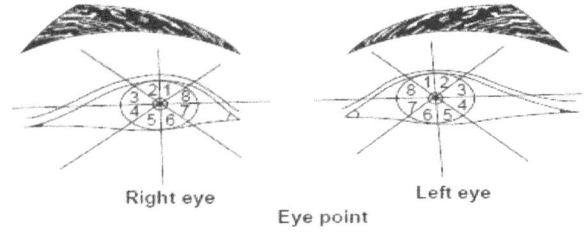

Right eye   Left eye
Eye point

1. Fei Dachang (Lung and large intestine)
2. Shen Pangguang (Kidney and bladder)
3. Shangjiao (Upper Energizer)
4. Gandan (Liver and gallbladder)
5. Zhongjiao (Middle Energizer)
6. Xin Xiaochang (Heart and small intestine)
7. Piwei (Spleen and stomach)
8. Xiajiao (Lower Energizer)

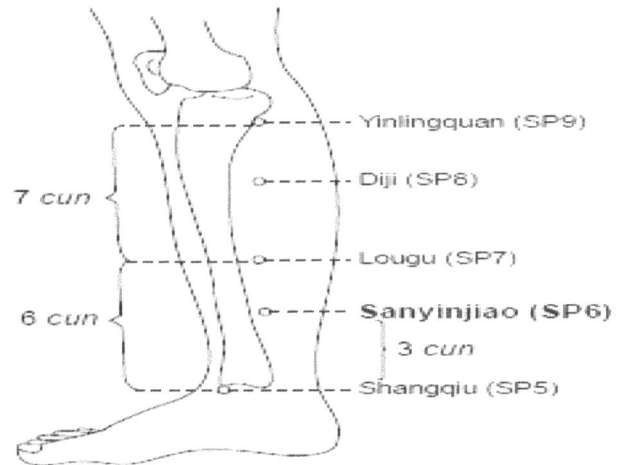

Yinlingquan (SP9)
Diji (SP8)
7 cun
Lougu (SP7)
6 cun
Sanyinjiao (SP6)
3 cun
Shangqiu (SP5)

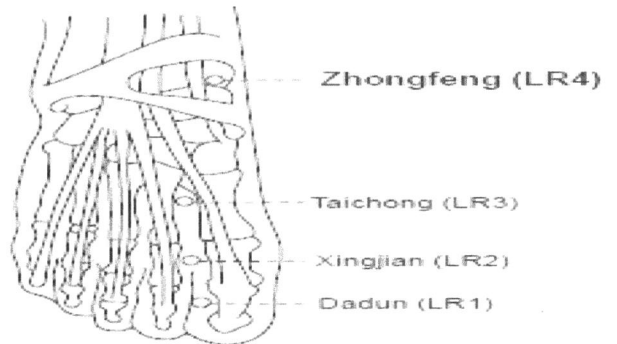

Zhongfeng (LR4)
Taichong (LR3)
Xingjian (LR2)
Dadun (LR1)

Cystitis

Taixi (KI3)–Sanyinjiao (SP6)

Acupuncture is performed. Insert the needles perpendicularly with strong stimulation. Leave the needles in place for 20–30 min.

Case: Ms. Li, a 58-year-old woman, felt a burning sensation during urination and suffered from frequent urination. She often had to get up during the night to urinate. She had a sensation of distention with pain in the lower abdomen. Urine analysis showed 1–3 red blood cells, 5–10 white blood cells, and proteinuria. She was diagnosed with cystitis. We treated her using this method. After one treatment, her symptoms were largely relieved. After two treatments, urine analysis showed 0–1 white blood cells, which means negative for white blood cells. She underwent a total of six treatments.

The bladder is located in the lower abdomen and stores urine. The bladder is the interior of the kidney. Diseases of the bladder are often caused by dysfunction of the kidney Qi transformation, which can cause problems with the bladder transforming Qi. Therefore, the Yuan Source point of the kidney meridian, Taixi (KI3), and points of the Jueyin channel, Sanyinjiao (SP6), were selected.

Cystitis

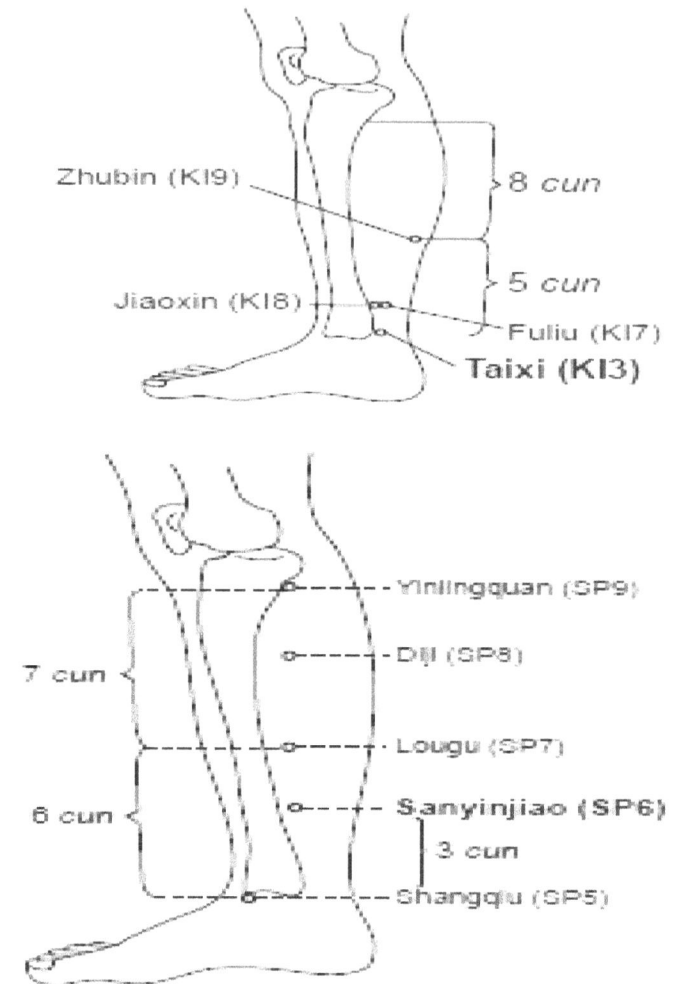

Guanyuan (CV4)–Shugu (BL65)

Acupuncture is performed according to the patient's reaction and situation. Usually, moderate stimulation is performed, without any specific needle technique. Insert a needle perpendicularly into the Guanyuan (CV4) at 1–2 *cun* deep. Then, insert the needles perpendicularly into the Shugu (BL65) on both sides at 0.8–1 *cun* deep.

Case: Coolman, a 20-year-old man, suffered from enuresis since childhood. The frequency of enuresis ranged from 1–4 times during the night. He felt tired and weakness in his lower back and extremities. The symptoms worsened after work. He passed clear urine in large amounts without urgency or a burning sensation. He tried herbal medicines from Chinatown, but they were not effective. We treated him with this method combined with herbal medicine. After one treatment, weakness in the lower back and extremities disappeared. After treatment for 1 month, the frequency of enuresis decreased.

Enuresis in Adults

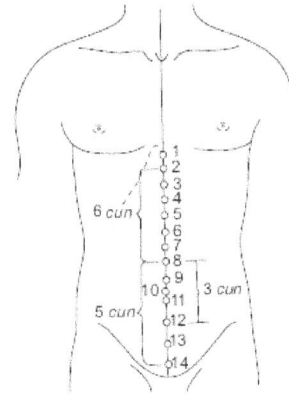

1. Jiuwei (CV15)
2. Juque (CV14)
3. Shangwan (CV13)
4. Zhongwan (CV12)
5. Jianli (CV11)
6. Xiawan (CV10)
7. Shuifen (CV9)
8. Shenque (CV8)
9. Yinjiao (CV7)
10. Qihai (CV6)
11. Shimen (CV5)
12. Guanyuan (**CV4**)
13. Zhongji (CV3)
14. Qugu (CV2)

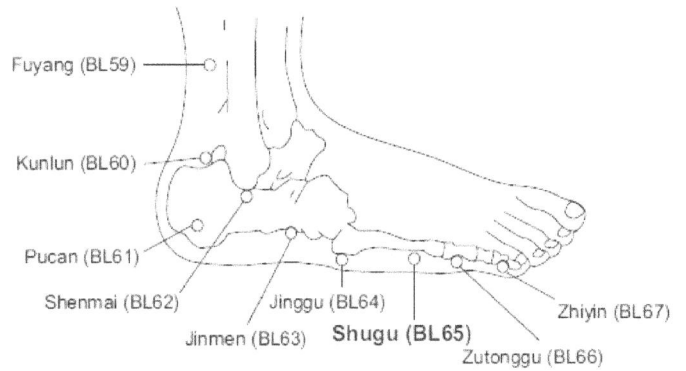

Fuyang (BL59)
Kunlun (BL60)
Pucan (BL61)
Shenmai (BL62)
Jinmen (BL63)
Jinggu (BL64)
Shugu (BL65)
Zutonggu (BL66)
Zhiyin (BL67)

Glomerulonephritis

Glomerulonephritis is referred to as edema in traditional Chinese medicine. Its treatment with acupuncture on paired points was first recorded by Gao Wu in the Ming Dynasty (1368–1644 A.D.) in his book Zhenjiu Juyin. He said that edema can be treated with acupuncture on the Fuliu (KI7) and if combined with acupuncture on the Shenque (CV8), it can be very effective. Edema can also be treated with acupuncture on the Yinlinquan (SP9) and moxibustion on the Shenshu (BL23).

Gan (Eye point)–Shen (Eye point)

Gan: Eye point located on the fourth area.

Shen: Eye point located on the second area.

Acupuncture is performed. Insert needles measuring (0.27–0.32) * 15 mm into the areas. After achieving the needle pricking sensation, leave the needles in place for 20–30 min.

Case: Mr. Caoqi, a 25-year-old Japanese man's urine had been the color of tea for 5 years, but he paid little attention to it. Three years ago, urine analysis showed protein ++ and a visual field during a microscopic analysis was full of red blood cells. Despite treatment at many clinics, the symptoms did not improve. After 10 treatments with this method, urine analysis results were normal.

Glomerulonephritis

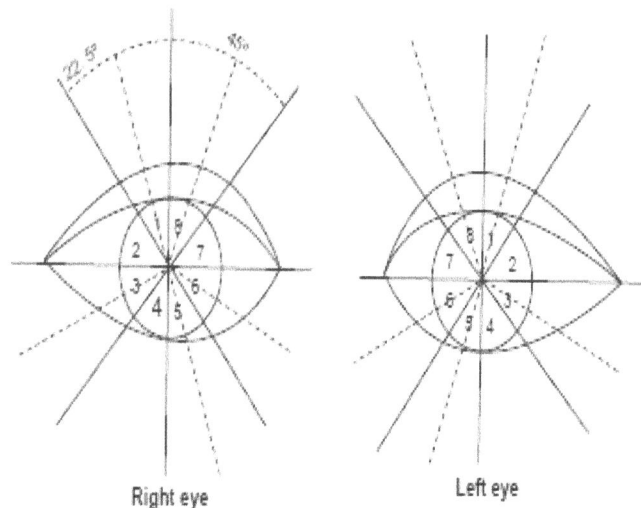

Right eye   Left eye

1. Shen Pangguang (Kidney and bladder)
2. Shangjiao (Upper Energizer)
3. Gandan (Liver and gallbladder)
4. Zhongjiao (Middle Energizer)
5. Xin Xiaochang (Heart and small intestine)
6. Piwei (Spleen and stomach)
7. Xiajiao (Lower Energizer)
8. Fei Dachang (Lung and large intestine)

Prostatitis

Prostatitis

Treatment of prostatitis with acupuncture on paired points was recorded by Wang Zhizhong in the Song Dynasty (960–1279 A.D.) in his book Zhenjiu Zishengjing. He said that the Zhongfeng (LR4) and Xingjian (LR2) could be used for treating shivering, white urine, and dysuria.

Waiguan (TE5)–Suliao (GV25)

Acupuncture is performed. Insert filiform needles into the points, performing the reducing needle technique. Leave the needles in place for 30 min.

Case: Mr. Ma, a 48-year-old teacher, had difficulty in urination for six months. He also experienced frequent urination, bloating, and excessive phlegm and used to masturbate. He took western medicine for some time, but the symptoms did not improve. We treated him with this method combined with administration of herbal medicines. After three treatments, his symptoms were relieved. After four more treatments combined with an abdominal breathing technique, he was cured.

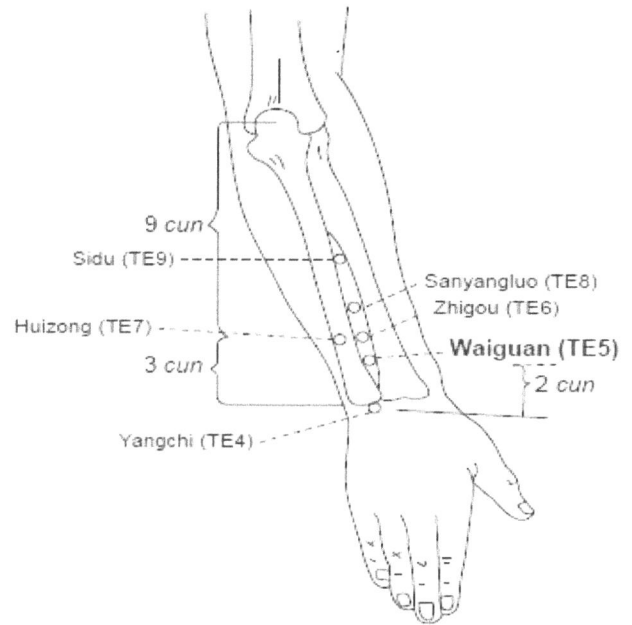

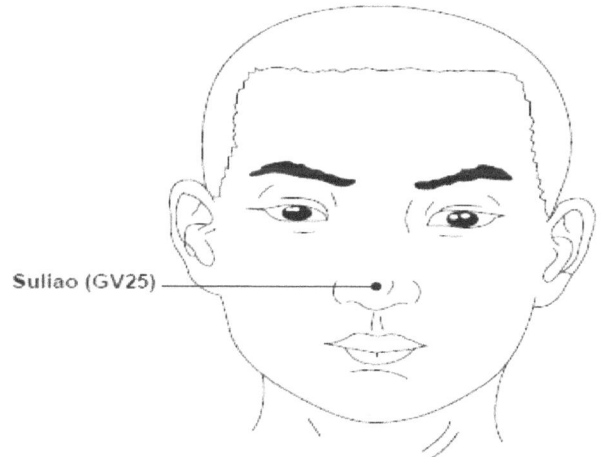

Enlarged Prostate

Shen (Eye point)–Gan (Eye point)

These two points belong to the eye points. Traditional eye acupuncture was established by Mr. Peng Jingshan in mainland China, who was my teacher. This eye point system is different from that of Tong's points.

Acupuncture is performed. Insert the needles into the Shen and Gan around the eyes. Avoid the eyeballs to prevent bleeding. Mainly perform the reinforcing needle technique.

We have used this method for treating urine distention caused by an enlarged prostate. After one treatment, the patient could urinate immediately.

This disease is caused by deficiency of the essence and blood and disorder of Qi movement in the bladder. The treatment should focus on reinforcing the liver and kidney and regulating Qi movement in the triple energizer. Therefore, these two points were selected and acupuncture was mainly performed with the reinforcing needle technique.

Enlarged Prostate

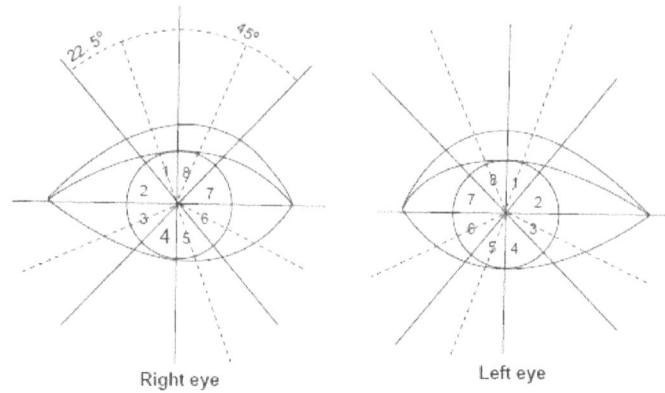

Right eye   Left eye

1. Shen Pangguang (Kidney and bladder)
2. Shangjiao (Upper Energizer)
3. Gandan (Liver and gallbladder)
4. Zhongjiao (Middle Energizer)
5. Xin Xiaochang (Heart and small intestine)
6. Piwei (Spleen and stomach)
7. Xiajiao (Lower Energizer)
8. Fei Dachang (Lung and large intestine)

102

Funiculitis

Funiculitis

Liukuai (1010.16)–Makuaishui (1010.14)

Acupuncture is performed. Insert the needles at 1–3 *fen* deep. My senior fellow Dr. Chen used this pair of points for treating funiculitis. The efficacy of this treatment was satisfactory.

Makuaishui (1010.14): Located at the lower border of the ala nasi, directly below the outer canthus.

Liukuai (1010.16): Located 1.5 *cun* lateral to the Shuigou (GV26), which is at the junction of the upper and middle third of the philtrum.

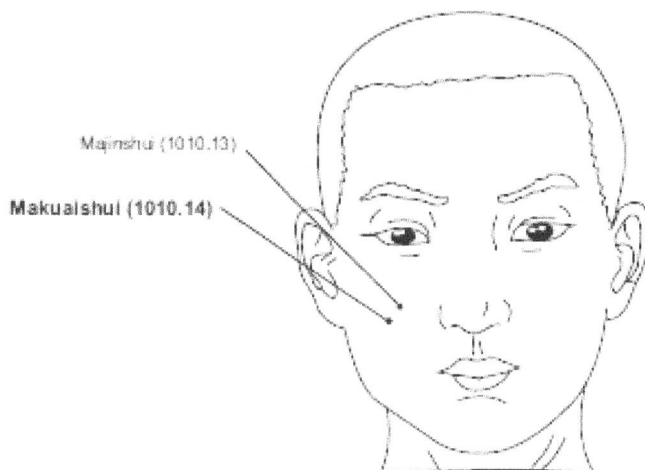

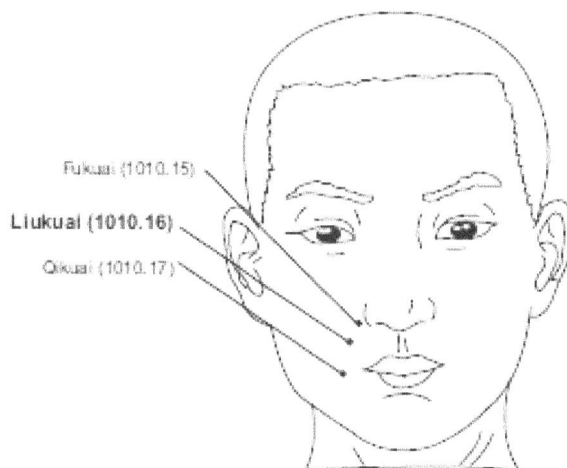

Hernia

Hernia can cause lower abdominal pain, which may radiate to the testis and cause swelling.

Baihui (GV20)–Dadun (LR1)

Acupuncture is performed. Insert the needles into the Dadun (LR1), which is located on the lateral side of the dorsum of the big toe, 0.1 *cun* posterior to the corner of the base of the nail.

Insert the needles, twisting and twirling at the same time, and performing the uniform reinforcing–reducing needle technique. Perform moxibustion until the hernial sac returns to the abdominal cavity. At the same time, massage the hernia sac to help it return. The effects can be observed immediately.

Hernia

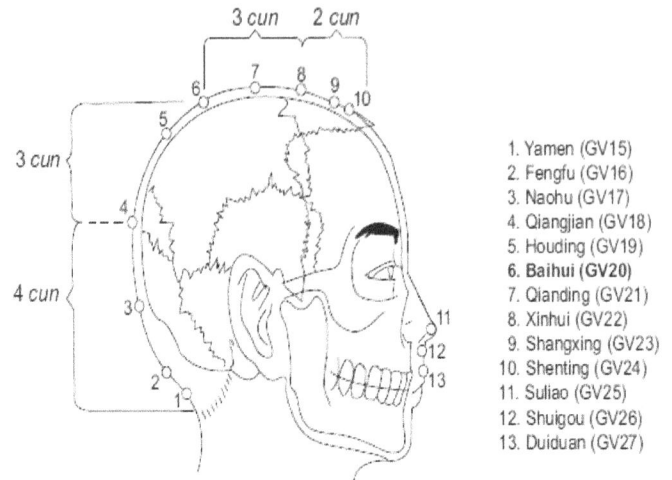

1. Yamen (GV15)
2. Fengfu (GV16)
3. Naohu (GV17)
4. Qiangjian (GV18)
5. Houding (GV19)
6. **Baihui (GV20)**
7. Qianding (GV21)
8. Xinhui (GV22)
9. Shangxing (GV23)
10. Shenting (GV24)
11. Suliao (GV25)
12. Shuigou (GV26)
13. Duiduan (GV27)

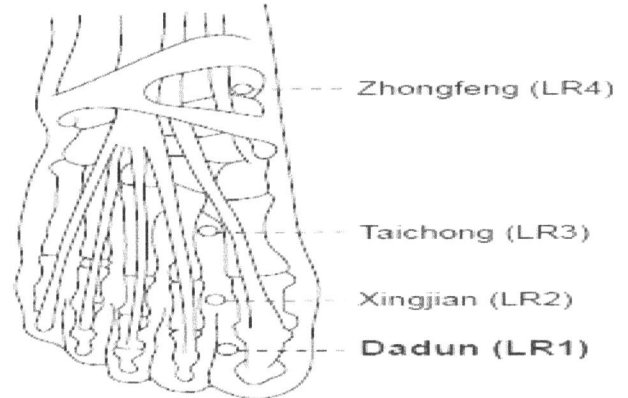

Zhongfeng (LR4)

Taichong (LR3)

Xingjian (LR2)

Dadun (LR1)

CHAPTER SIX

Diseases of the Nervous System

Neuropathic Headache

Headache is a common symptom of many acute and chronic diseases. It refers to pain occurring in the upper part of the head (the area above the eyebrows and occiput) due to stimulation of the sensitive tissue inside and outside the skull.

Xuanzhong (GB39)–Hegu (LI4)

Acupuncture is performed. The Xuanzhong (GB39) is located 3 *cun* above the tip of the external malleolus, on the posterior border of the fibula. Insert a 2-*cun*-long needle upward into the Xuanzhong (GB39) on the affected side. Perform the uniform reinforcing–reducing needle technique. Insert another needle at 45° obliquely upward into the Hegu (LI4). For patients who suffer from slight headache, the pain may stop immediately. For those who suffer from severe headache, acupuncture can be performed on the Taiyang (EX-HN5). Insert the needles obliquely on both sides.

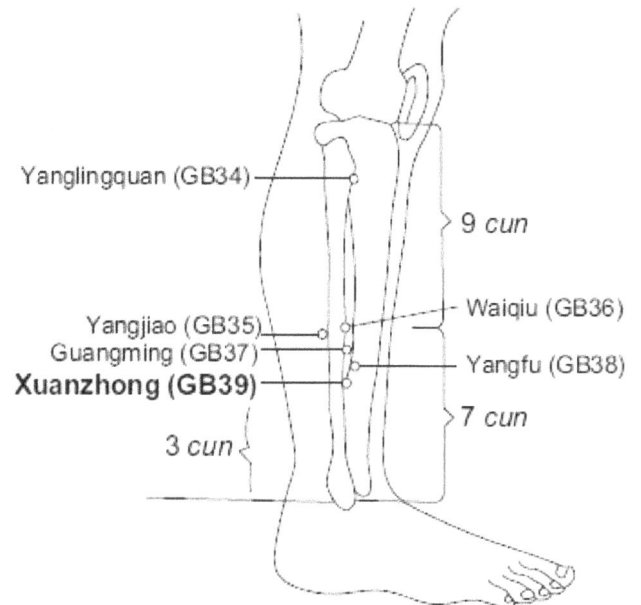

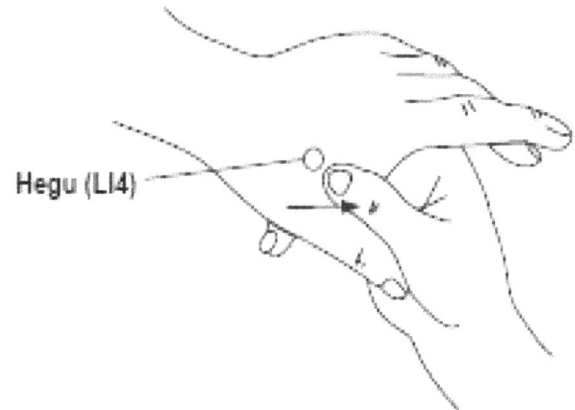

Trigeminal Neuralgia

Cesanli (77.22)–Sanzhong (77.05, 77.06, and 77.07)

Acupuncture is performed. Select the points on the unaffected side. Insert the needles perpendicularly. At the Sanzhong (77.05, 77.06, and 77.07), the needle pricking sensation will be very strong. Therefore, do not manipulate the needles on these points.

Case: Ms. Li, a 31-year-old woman, suffered from facial pain for 3 days. The pain worsened when she felt unhappy. The pain was so severe that she could not stay calm, eat, or even brush her teeth. We found that the pain was located on the left side of her face, which is dominated by the trigeminal nerve. We diagnosed her with trigeminal neuralgia and treated her with this method. After achieving the needle pricking sensation, the pain was immediately relieved. She received treatment twice a week. After 2 weeks, the pain disappeared completely.

Trigeminal Neuralgia

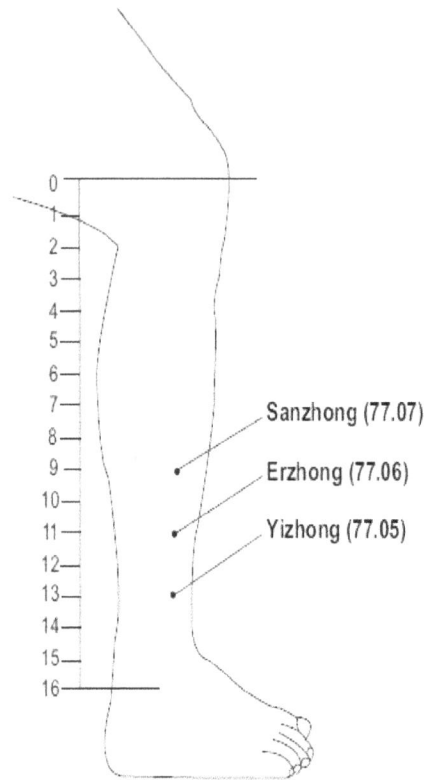

Sanzhong (77.07)
Erzhong (77.06)
Yizhong (77.05)

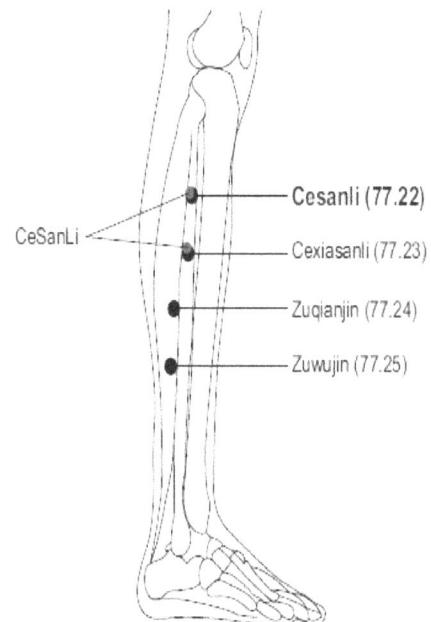

CeSanLi

Cesanli (77.22)
Cexiasanli (77.23)
Zuqianjin (77.24)
Zuwujin (77.25)

Facial Palsy

Facial Palsy

The treatment of facial palsy with paired points was applied relatively late in ancient times. It was first recorded by Wang Zhizhong in the Song Dynasty (960–1279 A.D.) in his book Zhenjiu Zishengjing. He said that the Jiache (ST6) and Quanliao (SI18) could be used for treating wry mouth and sensitivity to coldness. In the Song Dynasty (960–1279 A.D.), Yang reported in his book Yulongge that Dicang (ST4) and Jiache (ST6) can be used for treating a wry mouth. This pair of points was highly praised by many practitioners of later generations and is considered the most effective pair of points for treating facial palsy.

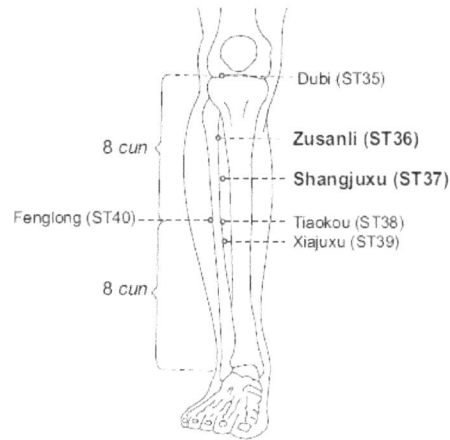

Formula One: Zusanli (ST36)–Shangjuxu (ST37)

Acupuncture is performed. Insert the needles into these points on both sides, performing the reducing needle technique, according to the direction of Qi movement in the channels. Leave the needles in place for 30 min.

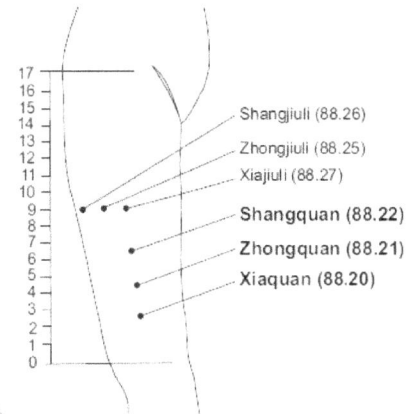

Formula Two: Sanchaer (22.16)–Sanquan (88.20, 88.21, and 88.22)

Acupuncture is performed. Select the points on the unaffected side. Insert a needle perpendicularly into the Sanchaer (22.16), performing the reducing needle technique. Perform bloodletting therapy on the Sanquan (88.20, 88.21, and 88.22).

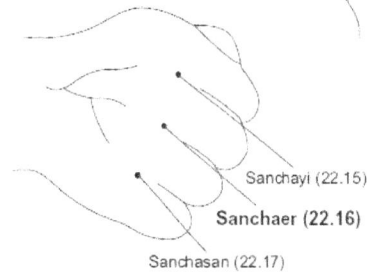

Case: Mr. Li, a 27-year-old, suddenly developed wry mouth and eyes without a known cause. He was unable to close his eyes completely, puff up his cheeks, or blow. We treated him with formula one three times, but the effect was not obvious. After that, we changed to formula two and cured him completely.

Facial Spasm

Upper 1 (wrist–ankle acupuncture)–Hegu (LI4)

Upper 1 (wrist–ankle acupuncture): Located on the palmar side of the wrist, between the ulna and tendon of the flexor carpi ulnaris.

Acupuncture is performed. Select the points on the affected side. After sterilization, insert filiform needles measuring 0.4 * 50 mm into the points. Leave the needles in place for 30 min. We used this method for treating facial spasm in one case. The symptoms disappeared after two sessions of treatment.

Wrist–ankle acupuncture is very effective in relieving various pain and injuries of the soft tissue. Hegu (LI4) is the Yuan source point of the hand Yangming channel. It can dispel Wind, relieve superficies syndrome, dredge channels, and stop pain.

Facial Spasm

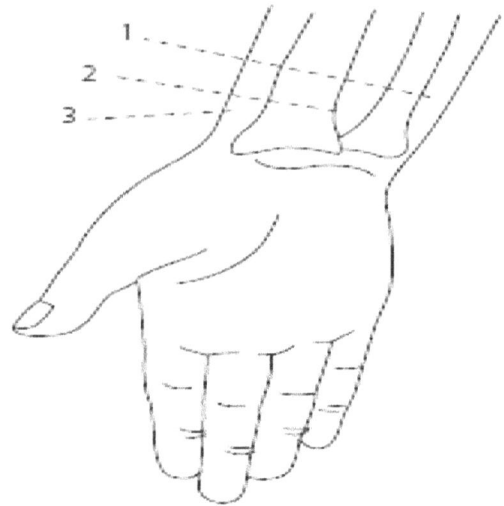

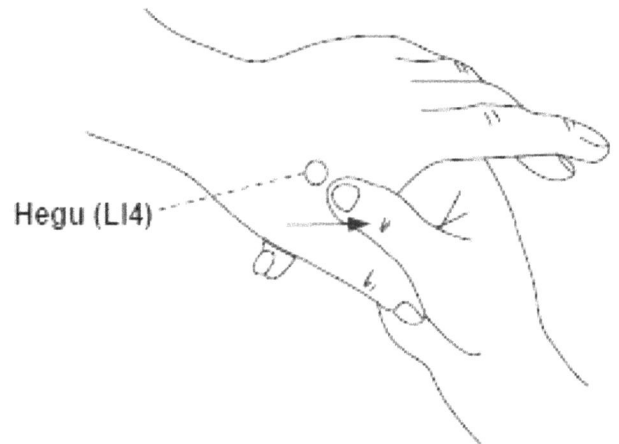

Supra-orbital Neuralgia

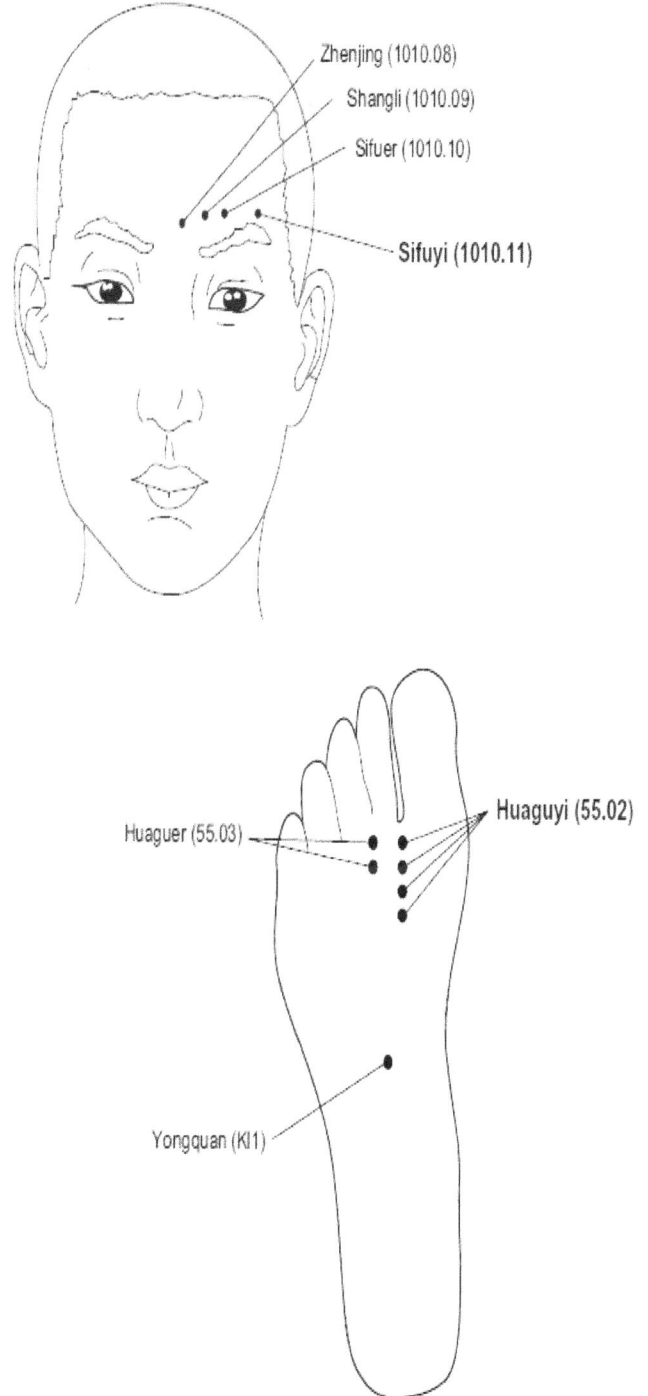

Supra-orbital Neuralgia

Sifuyi (1010.11)–Huaguyi (55.02)

Acupuncture is performed. Insert a 0.35 *15-mm needle into the Sifuyi (1010.11), penetrating the needle through the Cuanzhu (BL2). Insert a needle perpendicularly into the Huaguyi (55.02) 0.8–1 *cun* deep, without any specific needle technique. Usually, the pain will stop shortly after insertion of the needles. Treatment using this pair of points is learned from experience and is for your reference.

Case: Paul, a 40-year-old man, suffered from pain around the eyes and forehead for 3 years. The pain worsened during winter. He underwent many treatments without any effect. Examination: His visual acuity was 0.9. He had tenderness of the eyebrows, thin white tongue fur, and a tight pulse. We diagnosed him with supra-orbital neuralgia and treated him using this method. After one treatment, the pain disappeared and his visual acuity improved. After three treatments, all symptoms disappeared and his visual acuity became normal.

Zhenjing (1010.08)
Shangli (1010.09)
Sifuer (1010.10)
Sifuyi (1010.11)

Huaguer (55.03)
Huaguyi (55.02)
Yongquan (KI1)

Greater Occipital Neuralgia

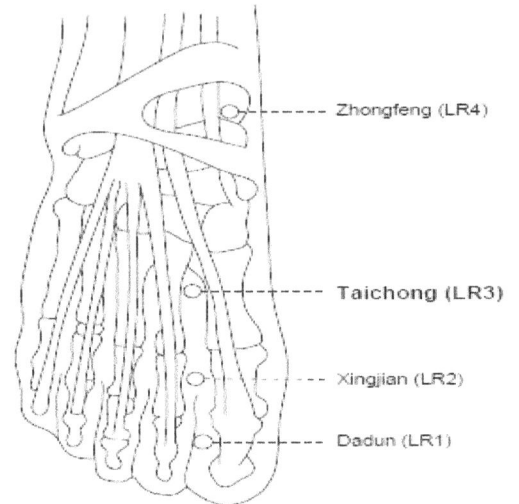

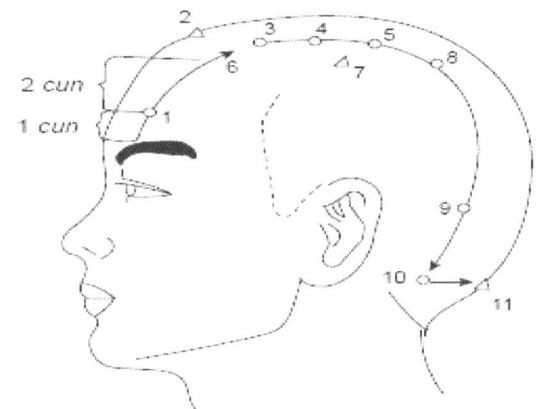

Greater Occipital Neuralgia

Greater occipital neuralgia refers to pain at the back of head and is quite common. Sometimes, the pain radiates to the top of head. This pain often worsens when moving the neck or coughing. It is usually caused by catching a cold. Usually, there is tenderness near the Fengchi (GB20).

Fengchi (GB20)–Taichong (LR3)

Acupuncture is performed. Insert the needles into the Fengchi (GB20), with the tips pointing in the direction of the apex of the nose. Insert the needles upward obliquely into the Taichong (LR3) at 0.8–1 *cun* deep. A better effect can be achieved by strong stimulation or electro-acupuncture.

Zhongfeng (LR4)

Taichong (LR3)

Xingjian (LR2)

Dadun (LR1)

2 cun
1 cun

1. Yangbai (GB14)
2. Shenting (GV24)
3. Toulinqi (GB15)
4. Muchuang (GB16)
5. Zhengying (GB17)
6. Benshen (GB13)
7. Touwei (ST8)
8. Chengling (GB18)
9. Naokong (GB19)
10. Fengchi (GB20)
11. Fengfu (GV16)

Obturator Neuralgia

Obturator Neuralgia

Ashi–Xuehai (SP10)

Bloodletting therapy is performed. After sterilization, prick three-edged needles into the points, letting the blood flow out. Next, press the points with clean cotton balls.

If the veins around the points are not obvious, massage around the points before pricking. If little amount of blood flows out, perform cupping therapy on the points.

This disease is caused by sudden sprain and contusion, which can affect the obturator nerve and induce inflammation. Qi and blood are stagnated. Stagnation can cause pain.

The Xuehai (SP10) is the main point for treating syndromes and diseases related to blood. A combination of acupuncture at the Ashi point and bloodletting therapy can dredge the channels, harmonize nutrient Qi and defensive Qi, activate blood, eliminate swelling, and stop pain.

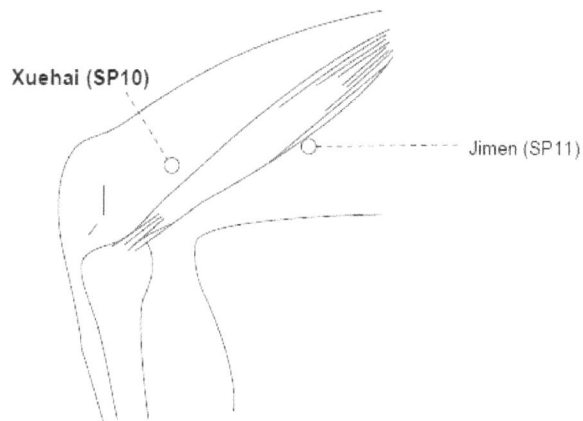

Xuehai (SP10)

Jimen (SP11)

Brachial Plexus Neuralgia

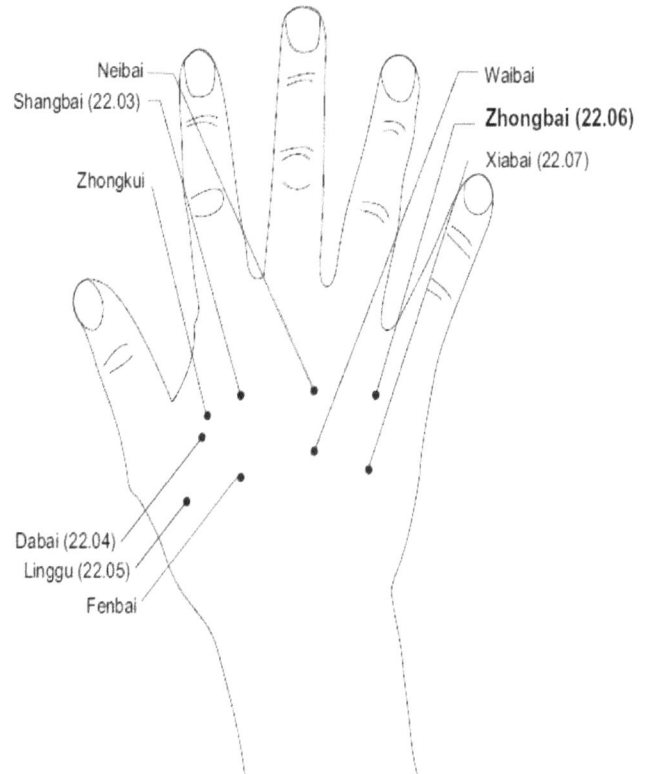

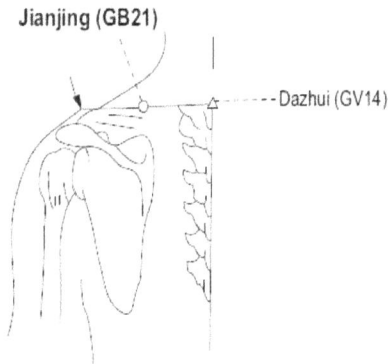

Jianjing (GB21)–Zhongbai (22.06)

Zhongbai (22.06): Located on the dorsal aspect of the hand between the ring and little fingers, 0.5 *cun* proximal to the base joints of these fingers (also termed as Guimen). Ask the patient to make a fist. Insert a needle into the Zhongbai (22.06) on the affected side at 3–5 *fen* deep. Insert the needles into the Jianjing (GB21).

The main symptom of brachial plexus neuralgia is pain. Based on the theory of traditional Chinese medicine, it is often caused by excessive wind and stagnation of blood. As the saying goes, stagnation causes pain and unblocking can stop this pain. Stabbing pain is usually caused by stagnation of blood. The Jianjing (GB21) is located above the supraclavicular and accessory nerves and posterior branch of the fourth cervical nerve. It can be used for treating pain and spasm of the muscles in the shoulders and back. The Zhongbai (22.06) is located above the dorsal digital nerve of the ulnar nerve. It is effective for relieving shoulder pain and numbness of the fingers. This method is more effective when combined with administration of the *Fuyuan Huoxue* decoction.

Intercostal Neuralgia

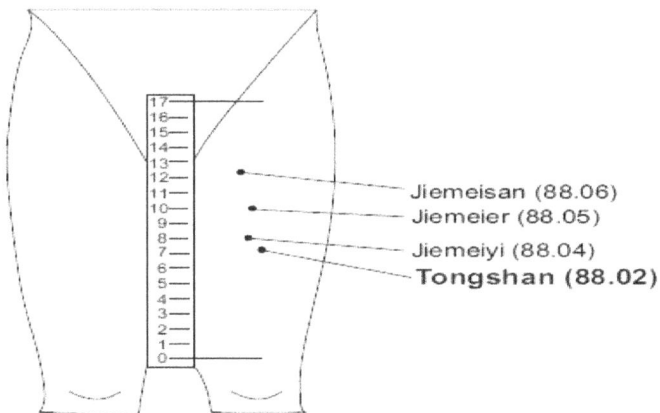

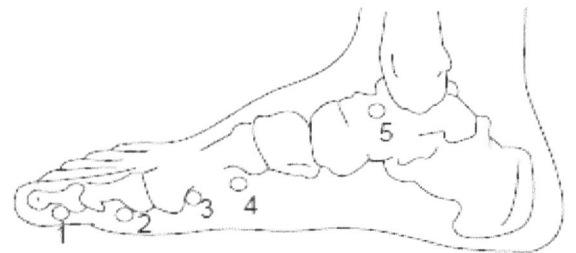

Formula One: Tongshan (88.02)–Xinchang (11.19)

Acupuncture is performed. Insert the needles obliquely into these points at 0.8–1.5 *cun* deep, without any specific needle technique. A good effect can be achieved with Mr. Tong's needle control method.

Formula Two: Neiguan (PC6)–Gongsun (SP4)

Acupuncture is performed. Insert the needles perpendicularly into these point at 1–1.5 *cun* deep, performing the reducing needle technique.

Experience: We used this pair of points for treating a patient who suffered from chest pain because of an injury due to falling. The pain was obvious when breathing in. After one treatment, the pain was relieved by approximately 80%. After two treatments combined with administration of herbal medicine, the pain disappeared completely.

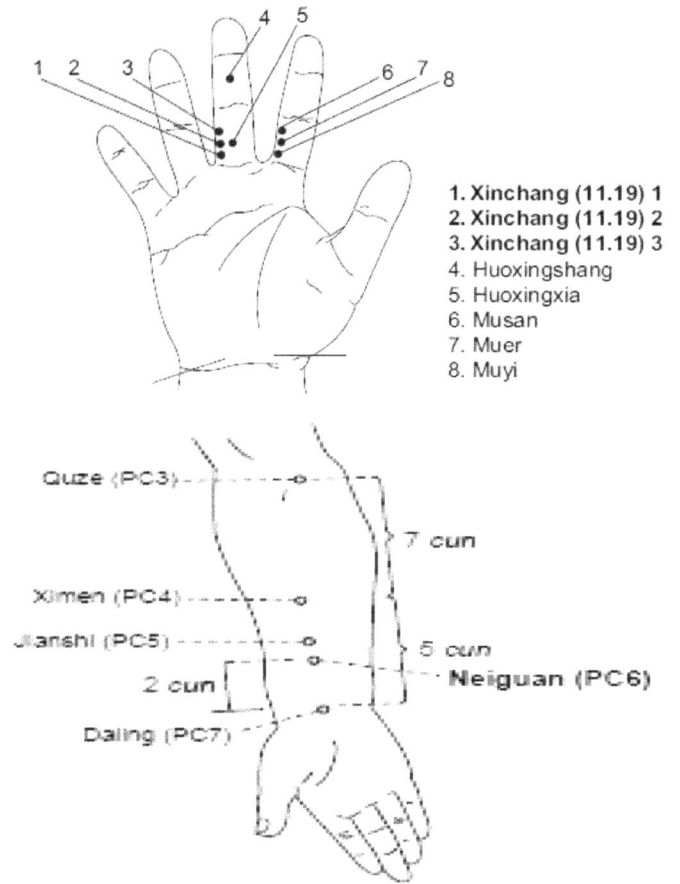

1. Xinchang (11.19) 1
2. Xinchang (11.19) 2
3. Xinchang (11.19) 3
4. Huoxingshang
5. Huoxingxia
6. Musan
7. Muer
8. Muyi

Intercostal Neuralgia

Jiemeisan (88.06)
Jiemeier (88.05)
Jiemeiyi (88.04)
Tongshan (88.02)

1. Yinbai (SP1)
2. Dadu (SP2)
3. Taibai (SP3)
4. Gongsun (SP4)
5. Shangqiu (SP5)

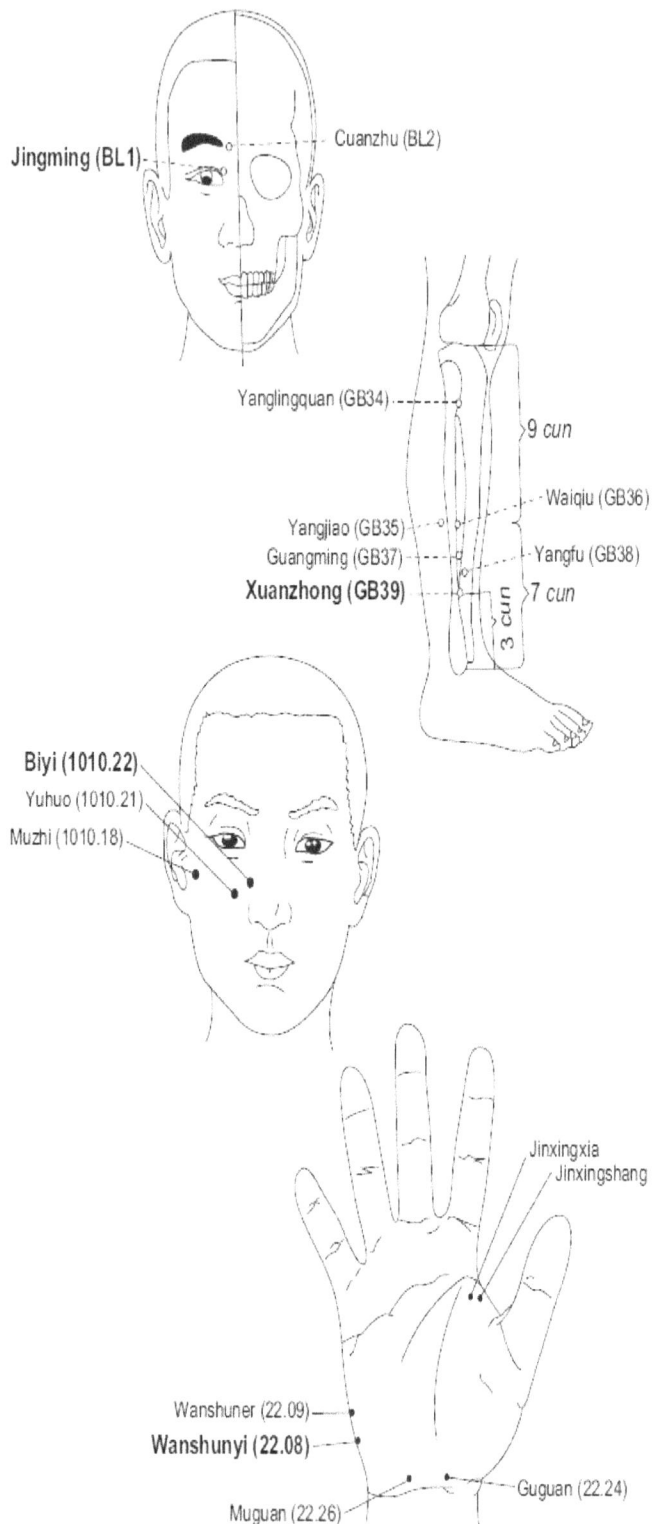

Sciatica

Sciatica

Sciatica refers to radiating pain along the sciatic nerve. It is a syndrome, not a single disease. There are many causes of sciatica, including lumbar disc herniation, vertebral column arthritis, and intraspinal tumor.

Formula One: Xuanzhong (GB39)–Jingming (BL1)

Acupuncture is performed. Ask the patient to lie on their back and close their eyes. Slightly press the eyeball and keep it at the outer canthus. Delicately insert a needle into the skin with the other hand. Next, insert the needle slowly to 0.8–1.2 *cun* deep. At the Xuanzhong (GB39), insert a 0.38 * (40–50)-mm needle at 1–1.5 *cun* deep. Perform the Dong-Qi technique. The treatment is immediately effective.

Formula Two: Wanshunyi (22.08)–Biyi (1010.22)

Acupuncture is performed. Inserting the needles into the Wanshunyi (22.08) along the bone at 1.5 *cun* deep can be very effective. Insert the needles obliquely into the Biyi (1010.22). Manipulate the needles for approximately 3–5 min.

Jingming (BL1)
Cuanzhu (BL2)

Yanglingquan (GB34)
9 *cun*
Waiqiu (GB36)
Yangjiao (GB35)
Guangming (GB37)
Yangfu (GB38)
Xuanzhong (GB39)
7 *cun*
3 *cun*

Biyi (1010.22)
Yuhuo (1010.21)
Muzhi (1010.18)

Jinxingxia
Jinxingshang

Wanshuner (22.09)
Wanshunyi (22.08)
Guguan (22.24)
Muguan (22.26)

Peripheral Polyneuritis

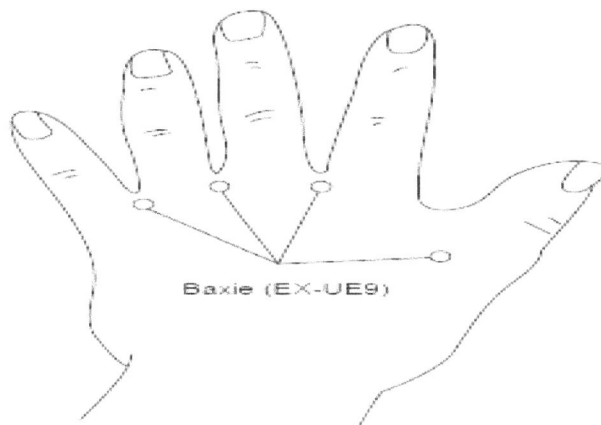

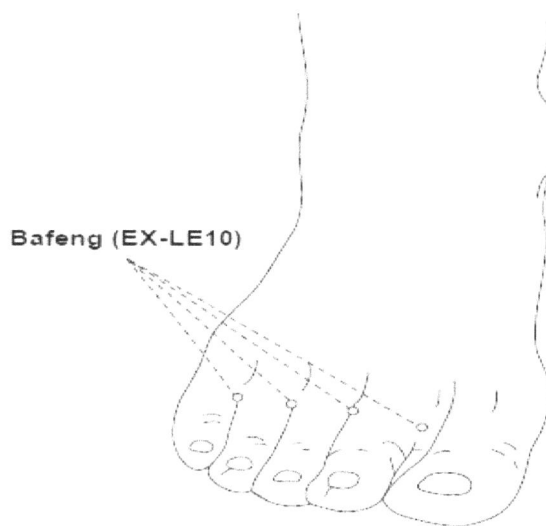

Peripheral Polyneuritis

Baxie (EX-UE9)–Bafeng (EX-LE10)

Bafeng (EX-LE10): Located on the dorsum of the foot, proximal to the margins of the webbing between all five toes, at the junction of the red and white skin. One foot has four points; both feet have a total of eight points.

Baxie (EX-UE9): Located on the dorsum of the hand, proximal to the margins of the webbing between all five fingers, at the junction of the red and white skin. Both hands together have a total of eight points.

Electro-acupuncture is performed. Insert the needles into the points on both sides, performing moderate stimulation. The needle pricking sensation will radiate to the tips of the fingers and toes. Connect the needle handles to the G6805 machine and choose a continuous frequency. The stimulation should be within the patient's tolerance.

Case: Mr. Wang, a 28-year-old dental technician, developed weakness and pain in his feet after sleeping on the floor overnight. At first, movement was not affected. A few days later, he felt stiffness in his feet while walking. The weakness in his feet worsened. At the same time, he developed weakness in his hands and had trouble making fists and straightening his upper extremities. After treatment with western medicine for several months, his condition did not improve. We treated him with this method. After 2 weeks of treatment, all symptoms completely disappeared.

Baxie (EX-UE9)

Bafeng (EX-LE10)

115

Radial Nerve Palsy

Yangchi (TE4)–Yanghai

Yanghai: An extra point located between the lateral epicondyle of the humerus and olecranon when bending the elbow.

Electro-acupuncture is performed. Insert 6-*cun*-long needles, performing the penetrating needle technique. Insert a needle into the Yanghai along the extensor carpi ulnaris. Insert another needle into the Yangchi (TE4) in the opposite direction along the extensor carpi ulnaris. Connect the needle handles to the electro-acupuncture machine and select dilatational waves. After 20 min, remove the needles.

Case: Jocy, a 29-year-old tooling worker, suffered from a sensation of electric discharge when straightening her right arm. The sensation radiated to her wrist and then to her little finger and ring finger. The symptom was relieved after rest, but resumed when she straightened her arm. She was introduced to our clinic by her neurologist. We treated her with this method, and she felt better after one treatment. After 1 month of treatment, the symptoms disappeared.

Radial Nerve Palsy

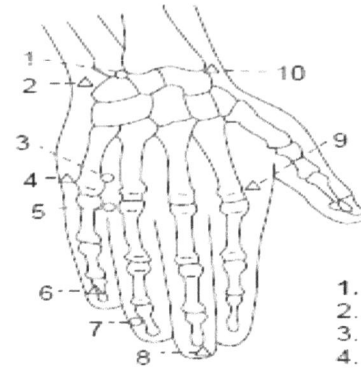

1. Yangchi (TE4)
2. Yanggu (SI5)
3. Zhongzhu (TE3)
4. Houxi (SI3)
5. Yemen (TE2)
6. Shaoze (SI1)
7. Guanchong (TE1)
8. Zhongchong (PC9)
9. Sanjian (LI3)
10. Yangxi (LI5)

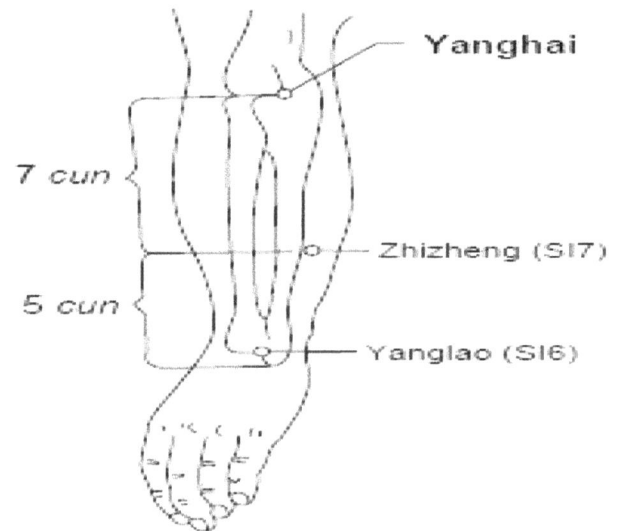

Yanghai

7 cun

5 cun

Zhizheng (SI7)

Yanglao (SI6)

Lateral Femoral Cutaneous Neuritis

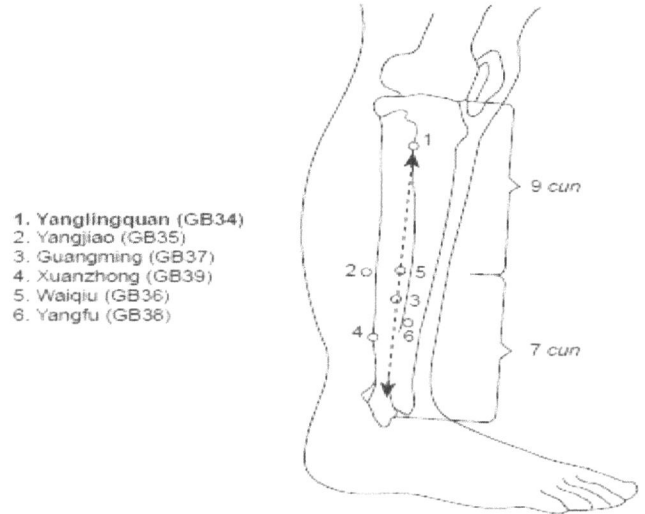

Lateral Femoral Cutaneous Neuritis

Yanglingquan (GB34)–Taichong (LR3)

Acupuncture is performed. Insert the needles perpendicularly into the Yanglingquan (GB34) at 1 *cun* deep, performing strong stimulation. Insert the needles into the Taichong (LR3) along the channel at 1 *cun* deep, performing strong stimulation.

Case: Scott, a 39-year-old man, suffered from numbness and tingling on the skin of his lateral right thigh for many years. His symptoms recently worsened, and he developed dysesthesia on the local skin. Despite treatment at many clinics, the symptoms were not relieved.

Examination: He had paresthesia in an area measuring 15 × 8cm on the lateral right thigh. There were no other abnormalities.

Diagnosis: Lateral femoral cutaneous neuritis. After one treatment session with this method, the skin sensation became normal.

This disease is caused by defense against coldness and dampness. Pathogens get into channels through the skin, blocking Qi and blood. The Yanglingquan (GB34) is located at the convergence of the tendon. It can be used to regulate Qi and blood in the lower extremities, relieve rigidity of muscles, activate collaterals, and nourish the channels.

1. Yanglingquan (GB34)
2. Yangjiao (GB35)
3. Guangming (GB37)
4. Xuanzhong (GB39)
5. Waiqiu (GB36)
6. Yangfu (GB38)

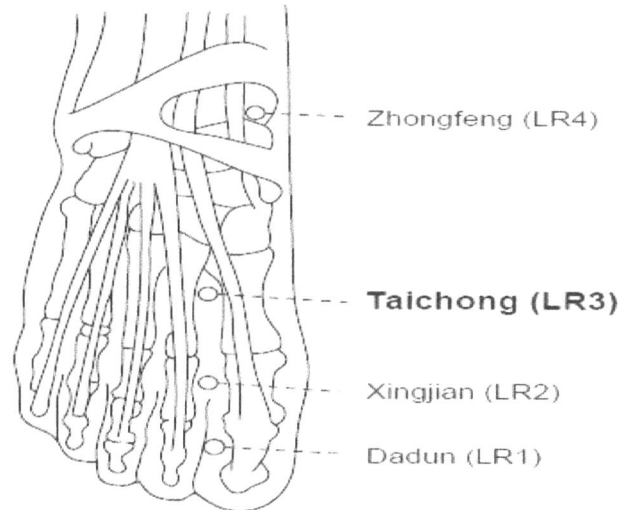

9 cun

7 cun

Zhongfeng (LR4)

Taichong (LR3)

Xingjian (LR2)

Dadun (LR1)

Gastrocnemius Spasm

Records on treatment of cramping with acupuncture were common in the Ming Dynasty (1368–1644 A.D.). For example, Li Ting recorded in his book Yixue Rumen that cramping of the legs and blurred vision can be treated with acupuncture on the Rangu (KI2) and Chengshan (BL57).

Sanyinjiao (SP6)–Chengjin (BL56)

Acupuncture is performed. Insert the needles into the Sanyinjiao (SP6) and Chengjin (BL56), performing the reducing needle technique. After achieving the needle pricking sensation, leave the needles in place for 30 min. During this time, manipulate the needles once every 10 min and perform moxibustion on the Chengshan (BL57).

Case: Mary, a 40-year-old woman, developed cramps of the right calf after moving to California and catching a cold 3 years ago. Cramping subsequently developed each time she caught a cold. The cramping occurred in each leg alternatively. At their worst, the symptoms occurred once a day for 3–7 days. She took western medicine and the cramping was relieved for 2 days, but it recurred. No positive signs were observed during physical examination. We treated her with acupuncture on the Sanyinjiao (SP6) and Chengjin (BL56) once a day for 5 days. The cramping did not occur during the treatment period. We taught her how to perform moxibustion herself. Subsequently, no recurrence of symptoms was noted.

Gastrocnemius Spasm

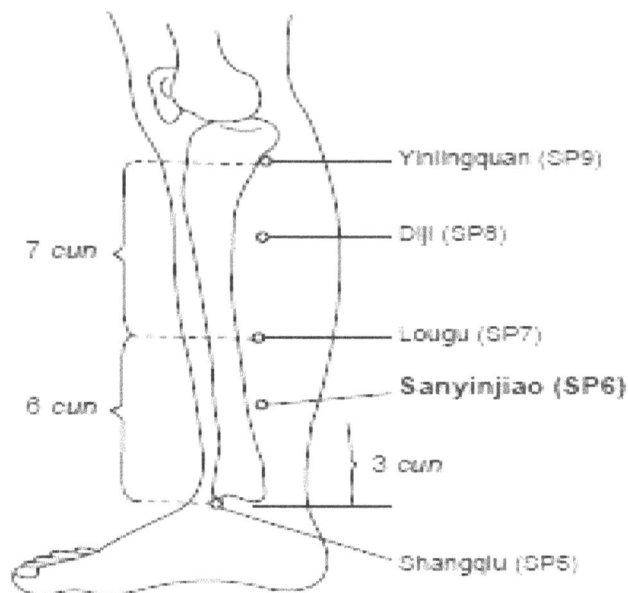

Yinlingquan (SP9)
Diji (SP8)
7 cun
Lougu (SP7)
Sanyinjiao (SP6)
6 cun
3 cun
Shangqiu (SP5)

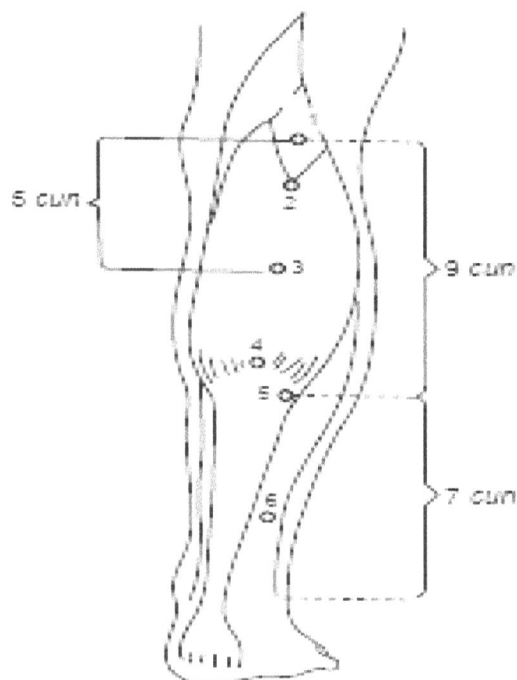

5 cun
9 cun
7 cun

1. Weizhong (BL40)
2. Heyang (BL55)
3. Chengjin (BL56)
4. Chengshan (BL57)
5. Feiyang (BL58)
6. Fuyang (BL59)

Peroneal Nerve Palsy

Peroneal Nerve Palsy

Tiaokou (ST38)–Taichong (LR3)

Electro-acupuncture is performed. Use 0.32 * (25–50)-mm needles. After sterilization, insert the needles obliquely into the Taichong (LR3), with the tip toward the big toes. Insert the needles into the Tiaokou (ST38) with the tip in the extensor hallucis longus. Connect the needles to the electro-acupuncture machine and turn it on. The big toes will move under electrical stimulation. Perform the treatment for 30 min each day for 2 weeks.

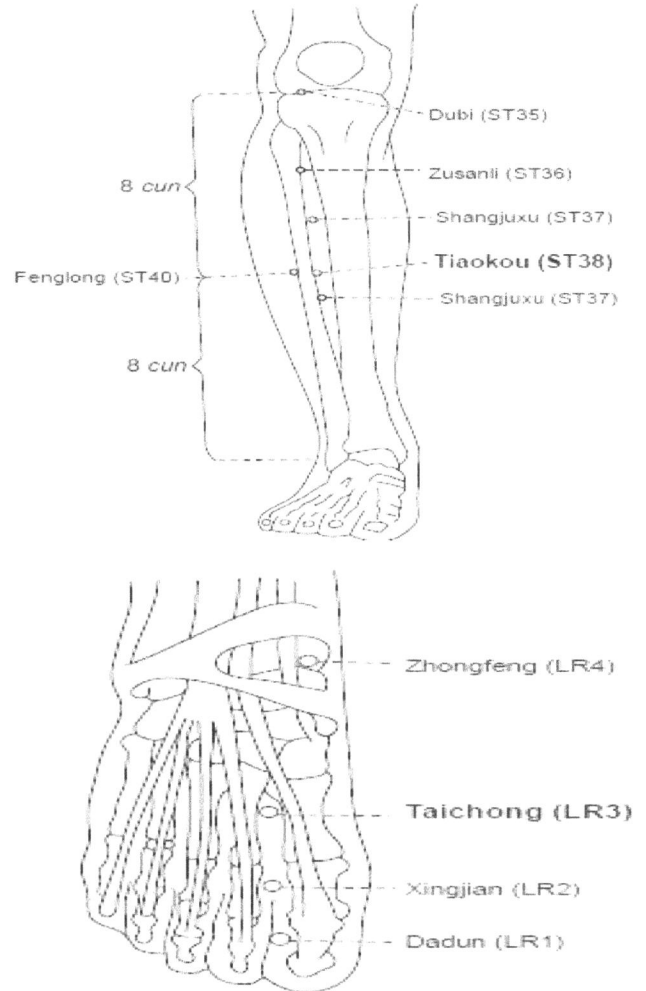

Spasmodic Torticollis

Formula One: Houxi (SI3)–Taichong (LR3)

Acupuncture is performed. After sterilization, insert 0.32 * 40-mm needles into these points, performing the Dong-Qi technique. The effect is extremely good.

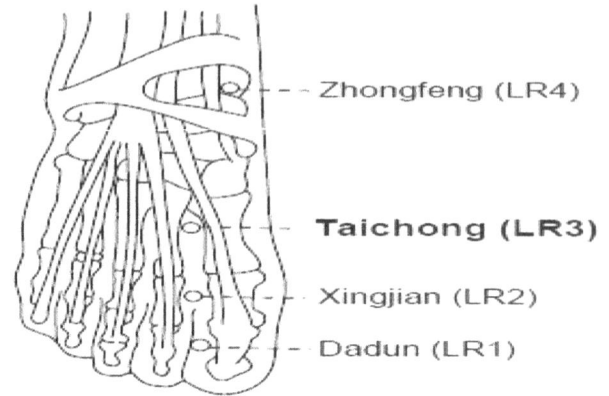

Formula Two: Jingqu (LU8)–Xuanzhong (GB39)

Acupuncture is performed. Insert the needles obliquely into the Xuanzhong (GB39) upward. Insert the needles obliquely into the Jingqu (LU8), with the tips penetrating the Lieque (LU7). This method is immediately effective in relieving pain.

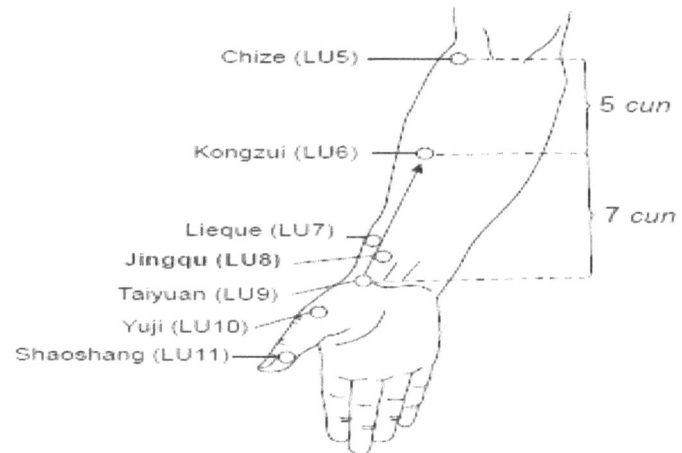

Spasmodic Torticollis

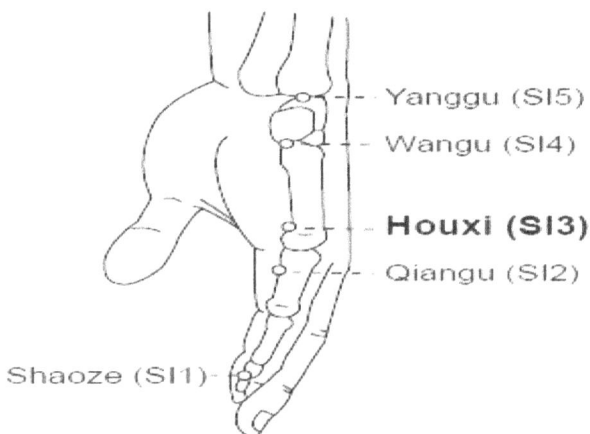

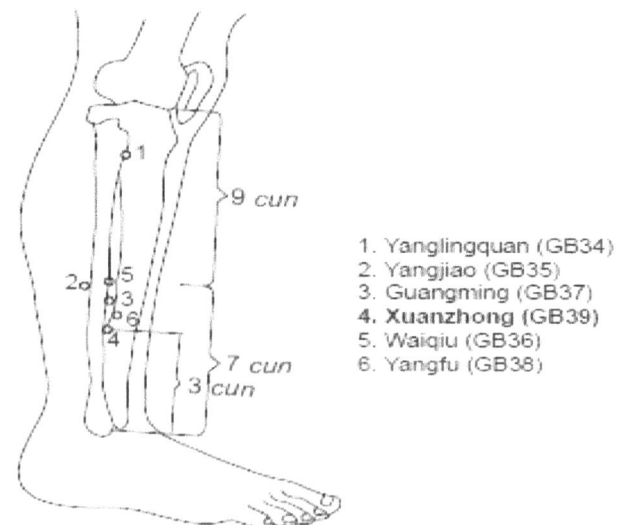

1. Yanglingquan (GB34)
2. Yangjiao (GB35)
3. Guangming (GB37)
4. Xuanzhong (GB39)
5. Waiqiu (GB36)
6. Yangfu (GB38)

Stroke

Stroke

Stroke is an emergency condition with symptoms of fainting, unconsciousness, wry mouth, trouble in speaking, and problems in moving one side of the body. It is usually caused by stagnation of Qi and blood, blocking of channels with phlegm and stasis, Yin deficiency of the liver and kidney, or hyperactivity of the Liver Yang.

Motor area (scalp acupuncture)–Leg motor and sensory area (scalp acupuncture)

Motor Area (scalp acupuncture): The upper point of the motor area is situated on the antero-posterior midline, 0.5 cm behind its midpoint. The lower point is the point on the temporal region where the supercilio-occipital line intersects the anterior hairline. The line connecting these two points is the motor area.

Leg motor and sensory area (scalp acupuncture). A line which is 3 cm long and parallel to the antero-posterior midline; its midpoint is 1 cm away from the midpoint of the antero-posterior midline.

Acupuncture is performed. After sterilization, insert the needles obliquely into the skin. After the tips reach a certain depth, increase the intensity of twisting and twirling to 220–260 times/min. Usually, after 1–2 min, the patient will have a needle pricking sensation in the limbs or organs. Continue manipulating the needles for 2–3 more min, then rest for 5–10 min. Manipulate the needles twice again then pause for 5–10 min. Perform the treatment once a day for 10 days. Normally, the symptoms can be improved in >90% patients.

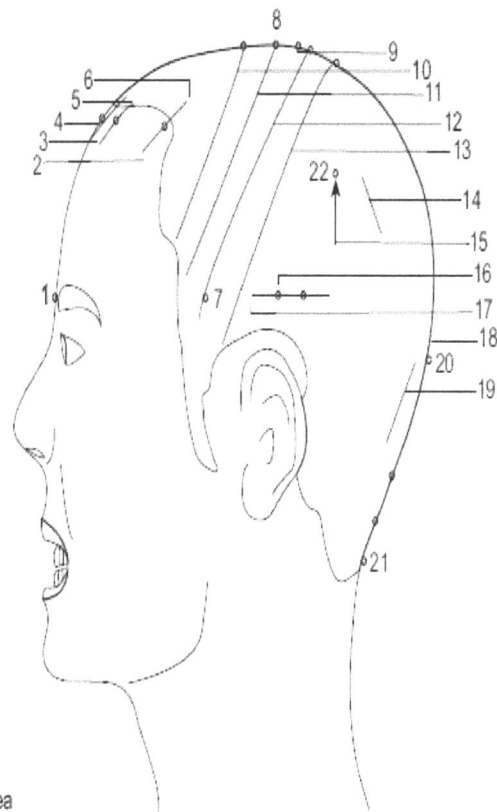

1. Glabella
2. Intestine area
3. Hepatocystic area
4. Thoracic cavity area
5. Stomach area
6. Reproductive area
7. Lower motor area
8. Midpoint of the antero-posterior line
9. Leg motor sensory area
10. Vasomotor area
11. Tremor control area
12. Motor area
13. Sensory area
14. 2nd speech area
15. Usage area
16. 3rd speech area
17. Vertigo and hearing area
18. Optic area
19. Balance area
20. Inion
21. Posterior hairline
22. Tubercle of parietal bone

Vertigo

Vertigo

Formula One: Hegu (LI4)–Taiyang (EX-HN5)

Taiyang (EX-HN5): An extra point located 1 *cun* lateral of the eyebrows and the lateral canthus.

Acupuncture is performed. Insert the needles into the Hegu (LI4) at 0.5–0.8 *cun* deep. Insert the needles into the Taiyang (EX-HN5) at 0.2–0.3 *cun* deep. After achieving the needle pricking sensation, perform the reinforcing needle technique. Leave the needles in place for 20 min.

Case: Ms. Wang, a 41-year-old woman, suffered from vertigo, distention sensation in the eyes, and nausea. The symptoms occurred 3–7 times a day and lasted for 40 min each time. After an episode, she felt weak, fatigue, chest tightness, shortness of breath, and a lack of appetite and had dull facial expressions. We treated her with this method four times. The symptoms disappeared completely.

Formula Two: Vertigo and hearing area (scalp acupuncture)–Quchi (LI11)

Vertigo and hearing area: A horizontal line that is 4 cm long and its midpoint is 1.5 cm above the apex of the ear.

Acupuncture is performed. Insert the needles into the points. Twist and twirl (200 times/min) the needles for 2 min. Pause for 10 min before resuming twisting and twirling the needles.

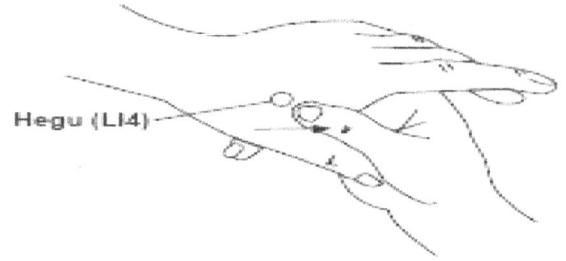

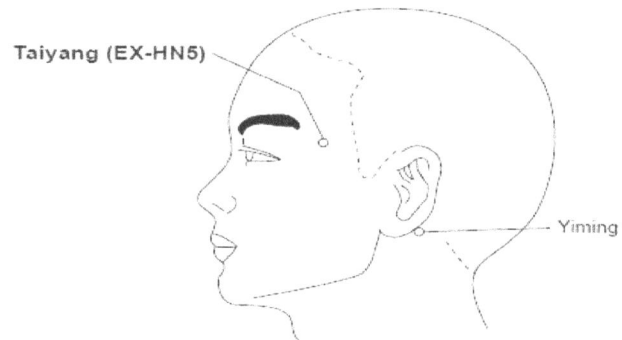

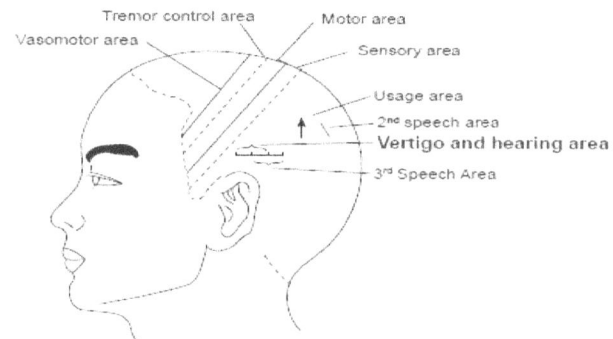

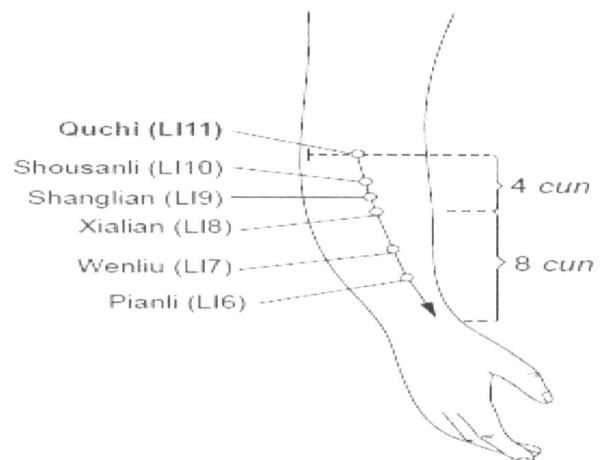

Migraine

Migraine

Migraine is a common symptom that is often seen in acute and chronic diseases. It refers to pain in the upper part of the head.

Formula One: Sizhukong (TE23)–Zulinqi (GB41)

Bloodletting treatment is performed on points on both sides. For acute symptoms, this method can be used to quickly stop the pain. It is more effective than acupuncture.

Formula Two: Sanchong (77.05, 77.06, 77.07)–Taiyang (11.23)

Acupuncture is performed. Taiyang, Dong's extra point, is located at the palmar side of the little finger, at the midpoint of the proximal joint. When performing Dong's needle technique on this point, 0.22 * 15-mm needles should be used. Perform the Dong-Qi needle technique.

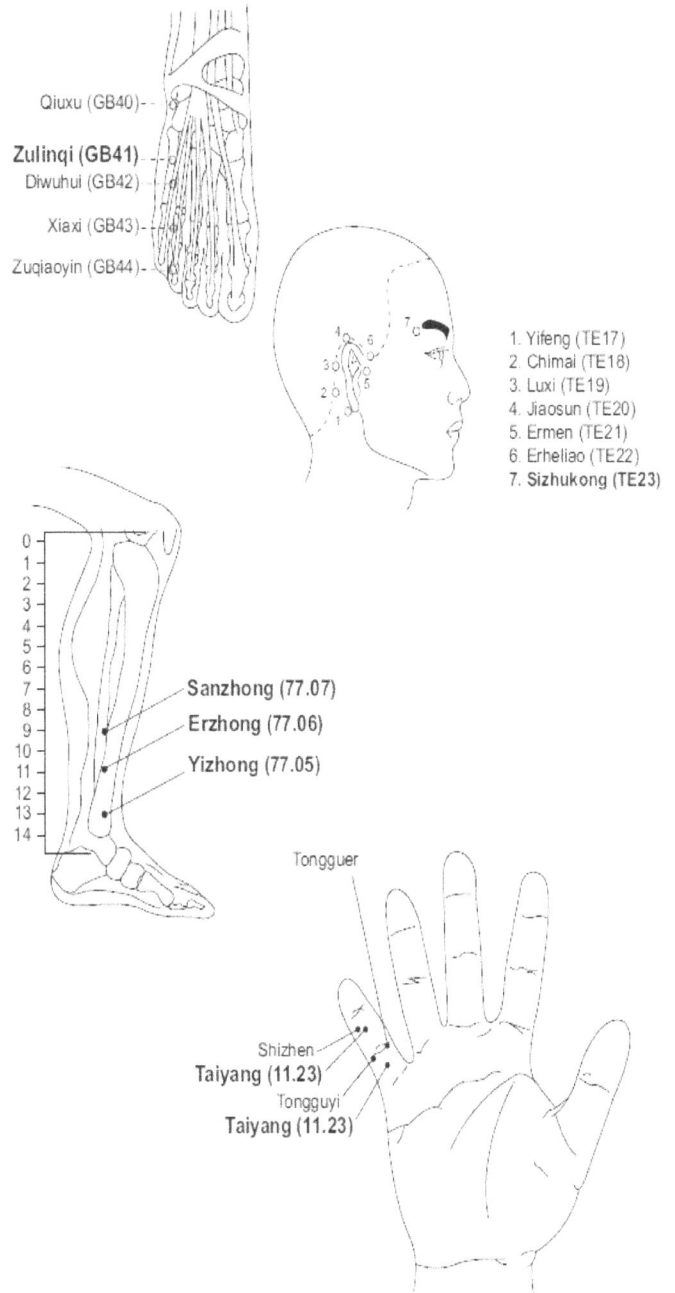

Qiuxu (GB40)
Zulinqi (GB41)
Diwuhui (GB42)
Xiaxi (GB43)
Zuqiaoyin (GB44)

1. Yifeng (TE17)
2. Chimai (TE18)
3. Luxi (TE19)
4. Jiaosun (TE20)
5. Ermen (TE21)
6. Erheliao (TE22)
7. Sizhukong (TE23)

Sanzhong (77.07)
Erzhong (77.06)
Yizhong (77.05)

Tongguer
Shizhen
Taiyang (11.23)
Tongguyi
Taiyang (11.23)

123

Sweating of Hands and Feet

Sweating of Hands and Feet

Formula One: Shenmen (HT7)–Neiguan (PC6)

Acupuncture is performed. Insert a needle into the Shenmen (HT7) with the tip penetrating through the Neiguan (PC6). Insert another needle into the Neiguan (PC6). Perform strong stimulation, then remove the needles. Perform this treatment every other day. In traditional Chinese medicine theory, sweat is the liquid of the heart. Shenmen (HT7) is the Shu-Stream point and the Yuan source point of the heart meridian. It can be used to calm the heart. Neiguan (PC6) is the Jing-River point of the pericardium meridian. It can be used for treating sweating.

Formula Two: Zhihan–Huoying (66.03)

When inserting a needle into the Huoying (66.03), you should be quick, precise, and resolute. Do not perform any needle technique. That is the key to using this point. Insert 0.20 * 50-mm needles perpendicularly at 1.5 *cun* deep. The patient will feel a sensation of electricity and numbness. For Zhihan, insert the needles obliquely at 30° with the tips upward. Do not twist the needles. We have used this pair of points for treating sweating, particularly sweating of the hands and feet. Usually, the effect is obvious after 5–10 treatments. The effect is comparable to that of endoscopic thoracic sympathectomy (surgery).

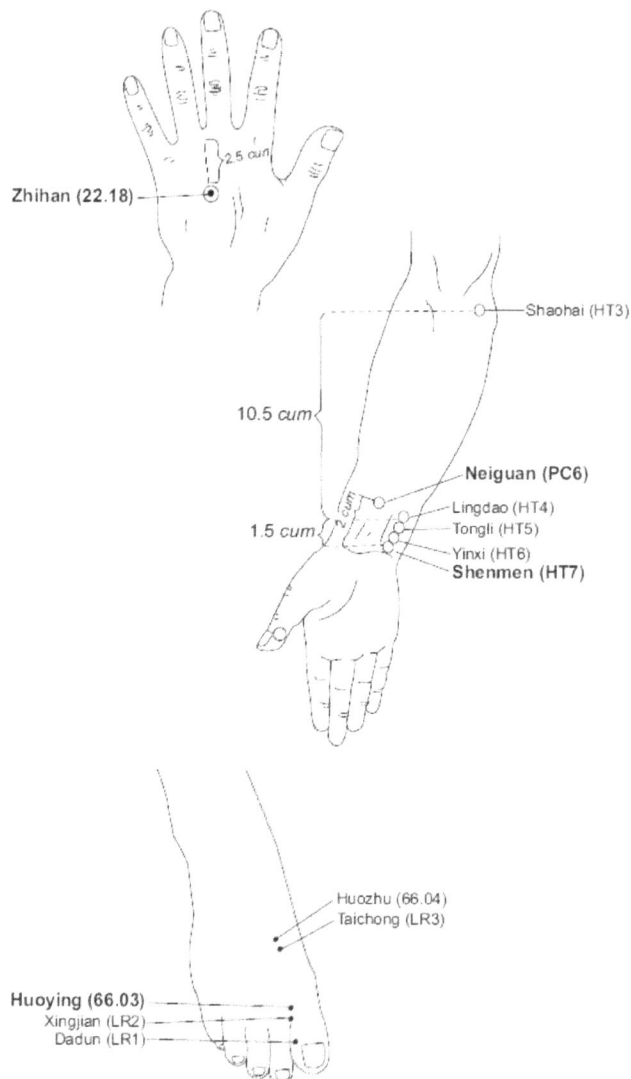

Myasthenia Gravis

Pi (eye point)–Shangjiao (eye point)

Pi (eye point): Consider the pupil as the center. Divide the area around the eye into eight zones. Give numbers to each zone, clockwise for the left eye and anti-clockwise for the right eye. The 7th zone is Pi.

Shangjiao (eye point): Divide the area using the above-mentioned method. The 3rd zone is Shangjiao.

After sterilization, press the eyeball slightly with the left hand and insert 0.32 * 15-mm needles into the Pi and Shangjiao. Leave the needles in place for 10–20 min, without any specific needle technique.

We successfully used this method for treating one case of myasthenia gravis.

Myasthenia Gravis

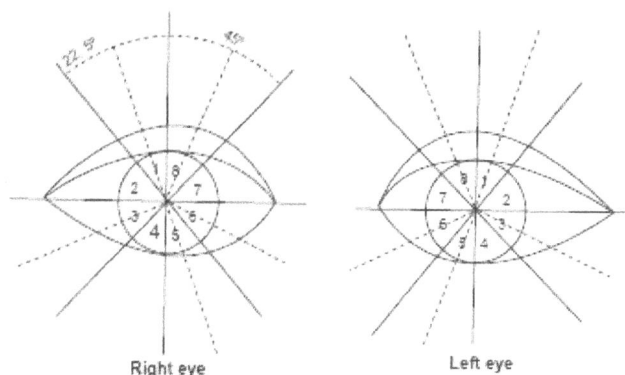

Right eye   Left eye

1. Shen Pangguang (Kidney and bladder)
2. **Shangjiao (Upper Energizer)**
3. Gandan (Liver and gallbladder)
4. Zhongjiao (Middle Energizer)
5. Xin Xiaochang (Heart and small intestine)
6. Piwei (Spleen and stomach)
7. Xiajiao (Lower Energizer)
8. Fei Dachang (Lung and large intestine)

Numbness in the Fingertips

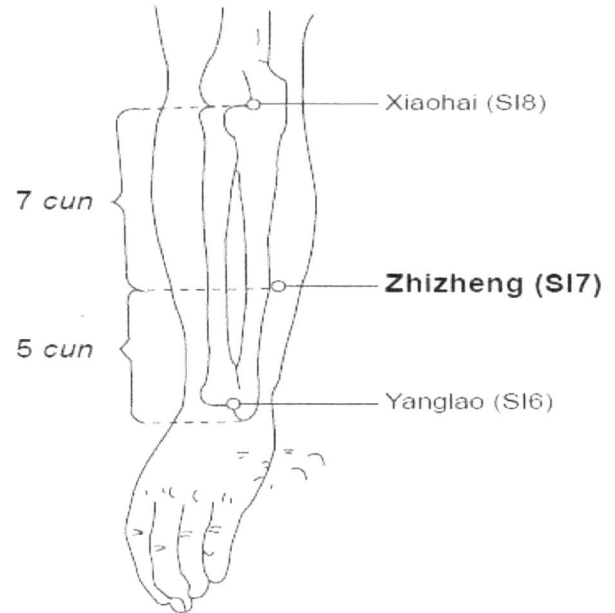

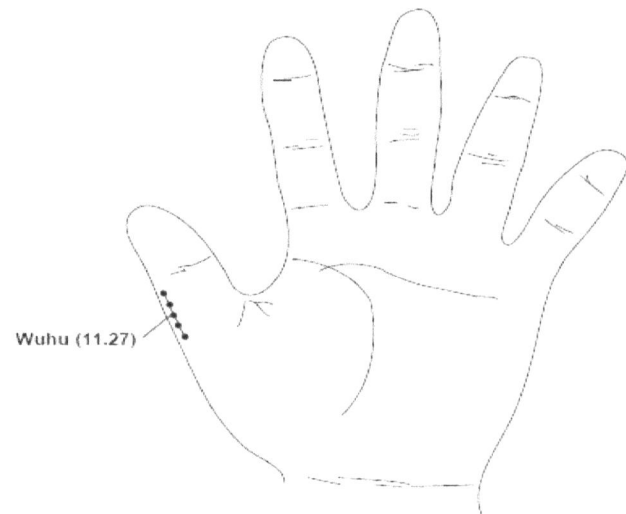

Numbness in the Fingertips

Zhizheng (SI7)–Wuhu

Acupuncture is performed. Wuhu is a set of extra points at the tips of the proximal joints of the index and ring fingers. Ask the patient to make a fist. Insert the needles perpendicularly into these points, performing the uniform reinforcing–reducing needle technique. Leave the needles in place for 20 min.

Case: Mr. Mucun, a 35-year-old man, suffered from numbness in the right thumb and index finger for approximately 1 year. Sometimes, his fingers were painful and he could not bend them or hold things. The pain sometimes radiated to his right elbow. He had a pink tongue with little fur and a fine rapid pulse. We treated him with this method for two sessions (six times). The numbness disappeared. He could bend his fingers again.

The Wuhu point mentioned here is not the same as the Wuhu (11.27) point in Dong's extra points. It is usually used to treat numbness in the fingertips and stomachache.

Paralysis

Motor area (scalp acupuncture)–Tremor control area (scalp acupuncture)

Motor area (scalp acupuncture): Located at the head and the temple, between the front Shencong and Xuanli (GB6).

Tremor control area (scalp acupuncture): parallel to and 1.5 cm anterior to the motor area. Electro-acupuncture is usually performed on this area.

After sterilization, insert 50-mm needles obliquely downward into the motor area on the unaffected side. When the needle is completely in the skin, except for its handle, insert another needle just under it. Insert another two needles into the tremor control area using the same method. Connect all needles with the electro-acupuncture machine. Turn on the machine, setting the frequency at 200–300 times/min. Leave the needles in place and keep the power on for 30 min. Perform this therapy once a day for 14 days. Pause for 1 week; then, resume treatment for 14 days. We have used this method for treating two patients with paralysis. One patient was completely cured, whereas the other patient showed improvement.

Paralysis

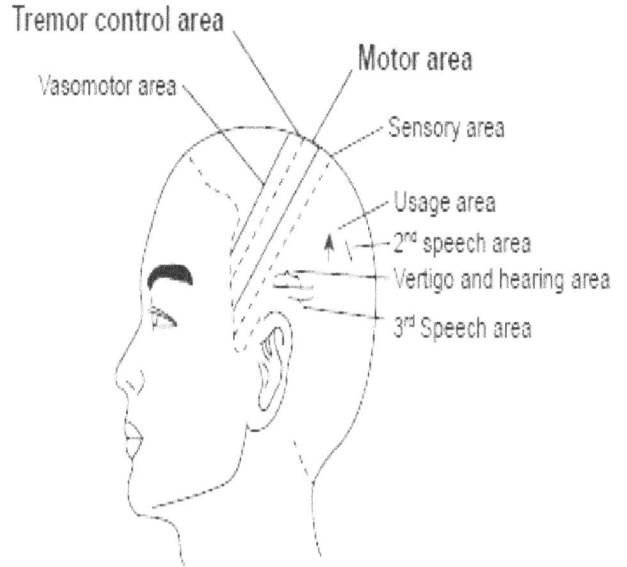

Tremor control area
Vasomotor area
Motor area
Sensory area
Usage area
2nd speech area
Vertigo and hearing area
3rd Speech area

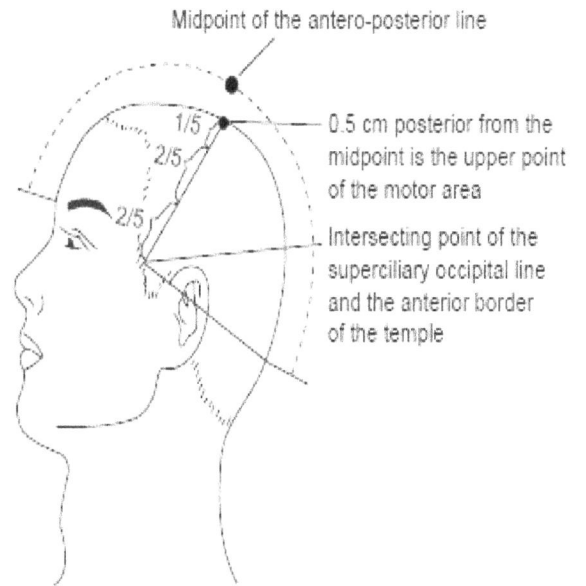

Midpoint of the antero-posterior line

1/5
2/5
2/5

0.5 cm posterior from the midpoint is the upper point of the motor area

Intersecting point of the superciliary occipital line and the anterior border of the temple

Aphasia

Aphasia

Yamen (GV15)–Zengyin

Zengyin: An extra point located on the neck at the midpoint of the line between the inferior thyroid notch and gonion.

Acupuncture is performed. After sterilization, insert the needles obliquely downward into the Yamen (GV15) at 0.5–1 *cun* deep. Then, insert the needles into the Zengyin, performing strong stimulation with twisting and twirling. Subsequently, remove the needles.

Case:

Ms. Mamei, a 82-year-old woman, developed aphasia after falling from a height and being struck on the face. We treated her with this method. After one treatment, she could speak again.

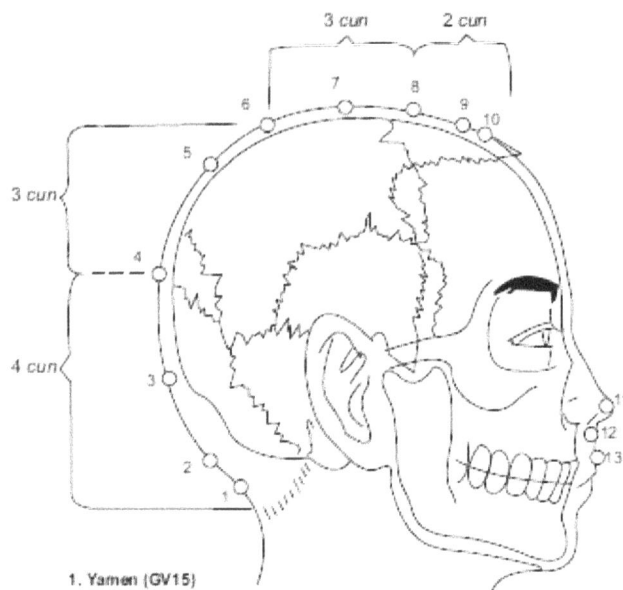

1. Yamen (GV15)
2. Fengfu (GV16)
3. Naohu (GV17)
4. Qiangjian (GV18)
5. Houding (GV19)
6. Baihui (GV20)
7. Qianding (GV21)
8. Xinhui (GV22)
9. Shangxing (GV23)
10. Shenting (GV24)
11. Suliao (GV25)
12. Shuigou (GV26)
13. Duiduan (GV27)

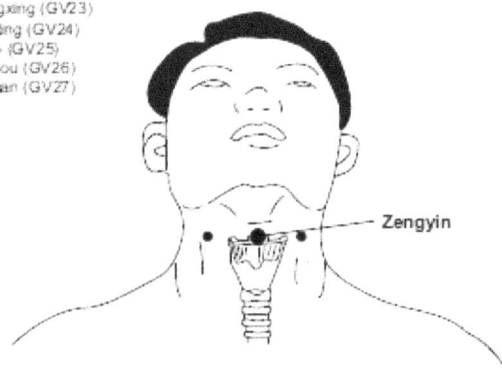

Zengyin

Insomnia

Formula One: Shenmen (Ear point)–Zusani (ST36)

Acupuncture is performed. Insert the needles into the Shenmen (ear pint) and Zusanli (ST36). After acupuncture, perform moxibustion.

Formula Two: Xiasanhuang (77.17, 77.19, 77.21)–Zhenjing (1010.08)

Acupuncture is performed. Insert the needles obliquely into the Xiasanhuang (77.17, 77.19, and 77.21) and Zhenjing (1010.08), without performing the needle technique. Insert the needles into Zhenjing (1010.08) at approximately 0.5 *fen* deep. Leave the needles in place for 20–30 min.

We have successfully used Formula Two for treating many patients with insomnia. This is for your reference.

Insomnia

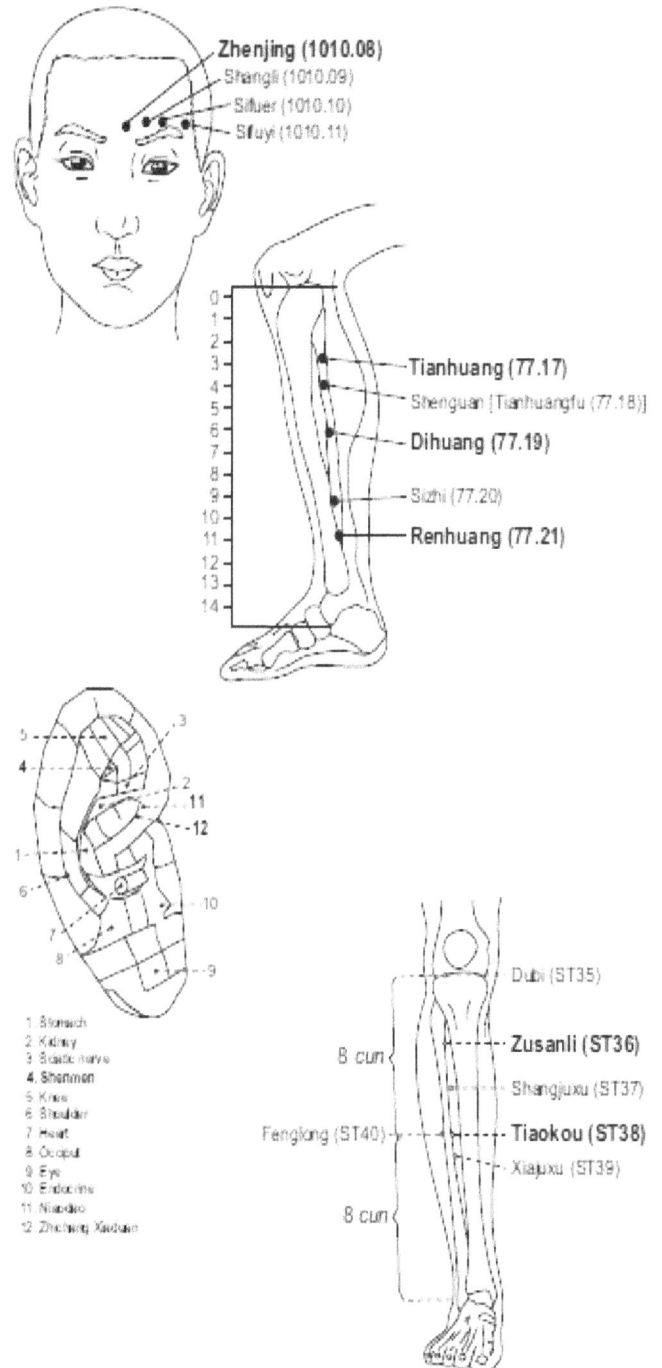

Neurosis

Neurosis

Ximen (PC4)–Shuigou (GV26)

Acupuncture is performed. Insert the needles perpendicularly into the Ximen (PC4) at 0.8–1.2 *cun* deep. Insert a needle 75° obliquely and deeply into the Shuigou (GV26), with the tip of the needle pointing to the nasal septum. Perform the reducing needle technique. Leave the needles in place for 30 min.

We have effectively used this method for treating five patients with neurosis.

In practice, the key is to radiate the needle pricking sensation to the elbow and upper chest when inserting needles into the Ximen (PC4).

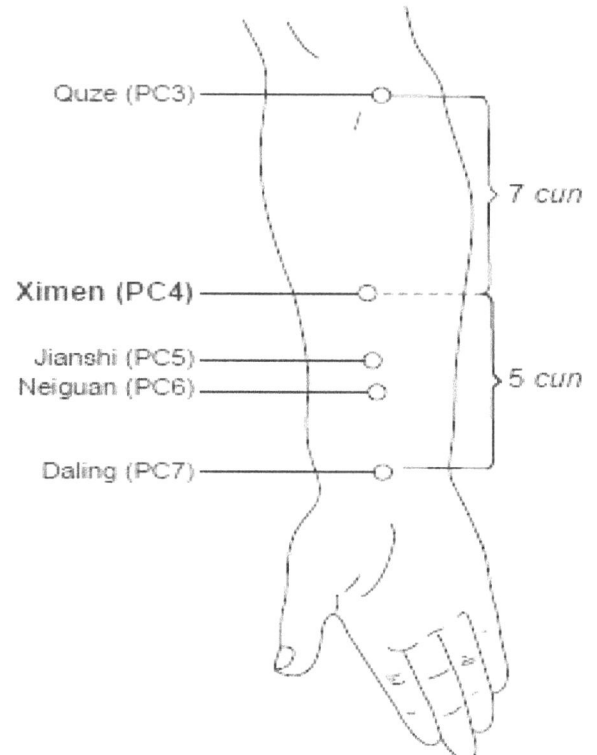

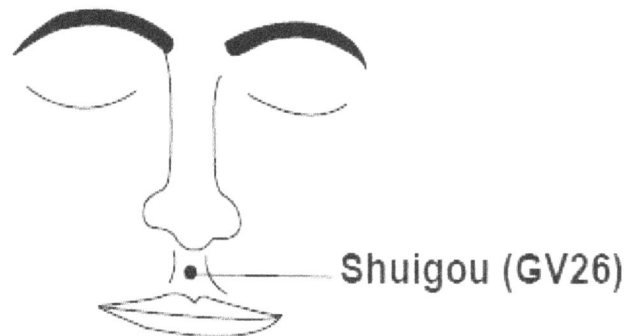

Chapter Seven

Gynecological Diseases

Dysfunctional Uterine Bleeding

Dysfunctional uterine bleeding is referred to as metrorrhagia or metrostaxis in traditional Chinese medicine. It is caused by chronic hormonal disorders and presents as hyperplasia or mixed endometrial changes on pathological examination from diagnostic curettage.

Formula One: Baihui (GV20)–Yinbai (SP1)

Moxibustion is performed. Ask the patient to lie on his/her back. Perform sandwiched moxibustion with pieces of ginger until the bleeding ceases, regardless of the number of moxa cones. Once the bleeding ceases, moxibustion is performed for an additional 10 min.

We have used this method to treat dysfunctional uterine bleeding in one case.

Formula Two: Huozhu (66.04)–Linggu (22.05)

The Huozhu (66.04) is located 1 *cun* above the Huoying (66.03). Acupuncture is performed on both these points, exerting an immediate effect. This is for your reference.

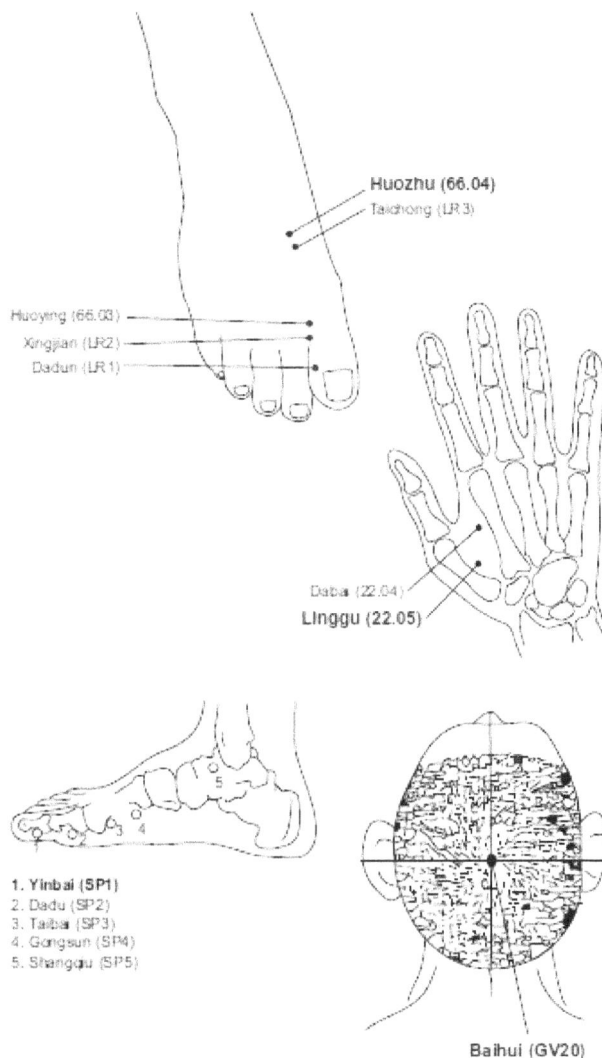

Huozhu (66.04)
Taichong (LR 3)

Huoying (66.03)
Xingjian (LR 2)
Dadun (LR 1)

Daba (22.04)
Linggu (22.05)

1. Yinbai (SP1)
2. Dadu (SP2)
3. Taibai (SP3)
4. Gongsun (SP4)
5. Shangqiu (SP5)

Baihui (GV20)

Menstrual Disorders

Menstrual Disorders

Treatment of menstrual disorders with acupuncture on paired points was recorded by Gaowu in the Ming Dynasty (1368–1644 A.D.) in his book Zhenjiu Juyin. Gaowu reported that menstrual disorders can be treated with acupuncture on the Diji (SP8) paired with the Xuehai (SP10) and on the Tianshu (ST25) paired with the Tianquan (PC2).

Xiasanhuang (77.17, 77.19, and 77.21)–Fuke (11.24)

Acupuncture is performed by inserting the needles perpendicularly into the Xiasanhuang (77.17, 77.19, and 77.21) at 1.5 *cun* deep and into the Fuke (11.24). These points are usually used for effectively treating menstrual disorders in women.

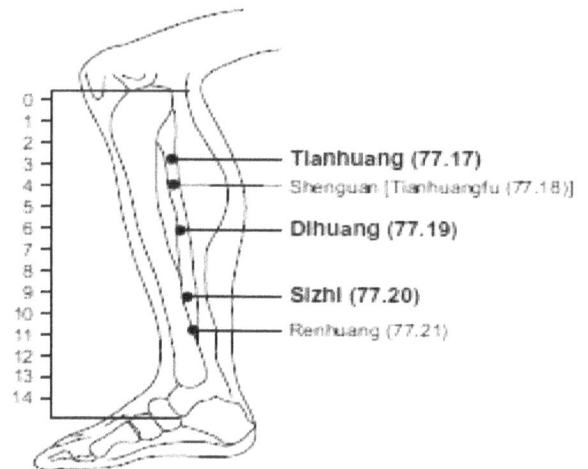

Tianhuang (77.17)
Shenguan [Tianhuangfu (77.18)]
Dihuang (77.19)
Sizhi (77.20)
Renhuang (77.21)

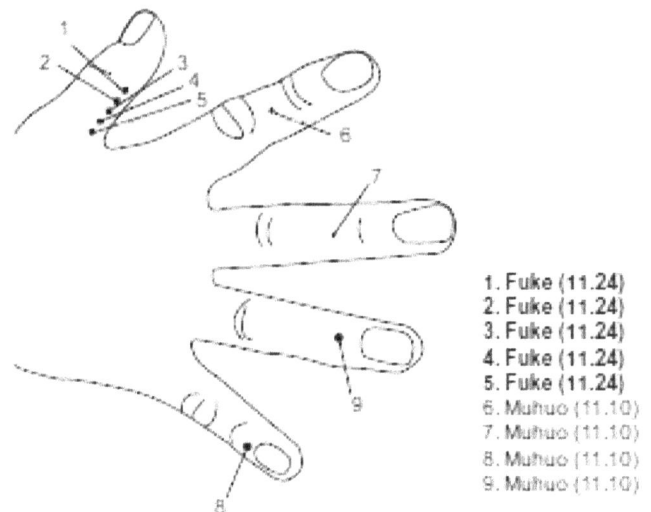

1. Fuke (11.24)
2. Fuke (11.24)
3. Fuke (11.24)
4. Fuke (11.24)
5. Fuke (11.24)
6. Muhuo (11.10)
7. Muhuo (11.10)
8. Muhuo (11.10)
9. Muhuo (11.10)

Dysmenorrhea

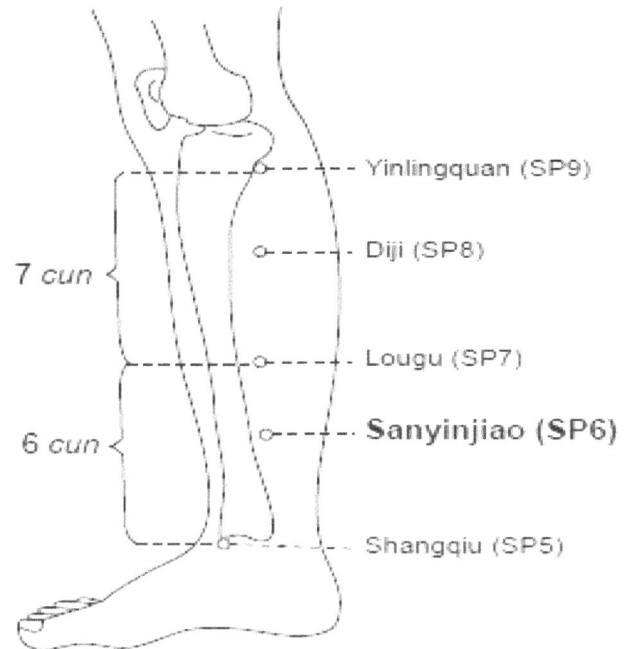

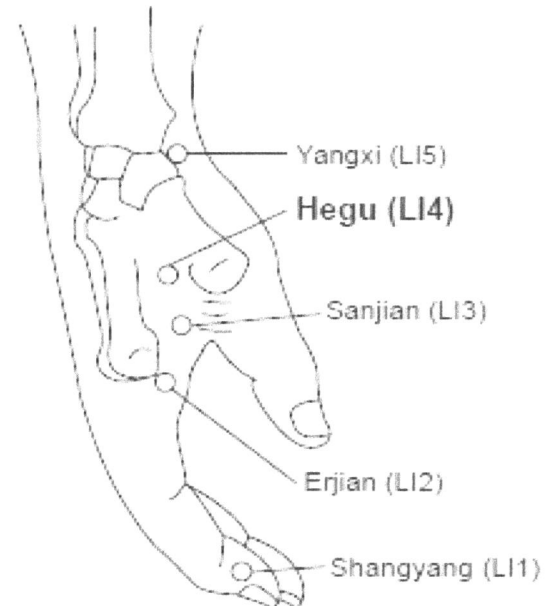

Sanyinjiao (SP6)–Hegu (LI4)

Acupuncture is performed. Ask the patient to lie on his/her back. After sterilization, insert 0.38 * 50-mm needles into the points, performing the uniform reinforcing–reducing needle technique. Leave the needles in place for 15 min. We have used this method to treat dysmenorrhea in one case.

Case: Ms. Zhang, a 24-year-old woman, suffered from dysmenorrhea. During her period, she felt pain in her lower abdomen and continued to be bent over at the waist and knees. She had a slow pulse. Pain was caused by cold coagulation and Qi stagnation in the uterus and we used this method to treat her. After one week, the pain had subsided and did not recur.

Given that the points on the left side govern blood and those on the right side govern Qi, their combination can be used for simultaneously regulating Qi and the blood. We used this theory to treat dysmenorrhea and successfully dispelled coldness.

Dysmenorrhea

Amenorrhea

Diji (SP8)–Neiting (ST44)

Acupuncture is performed. After sterilization, insert 0.27-mm needles into the points, by twisting them. After achieving the needle pricking sensation, leave the needles in place for 30 min. Perform the needle technique according to the syndrome: for deficient cold syndrome, needles are inserted slowly and twisting is maintained for 1 min and for excessive heat, needles are rapidly inserted and twisting is kept for half a minute before removing the needles.

Amenorrhea

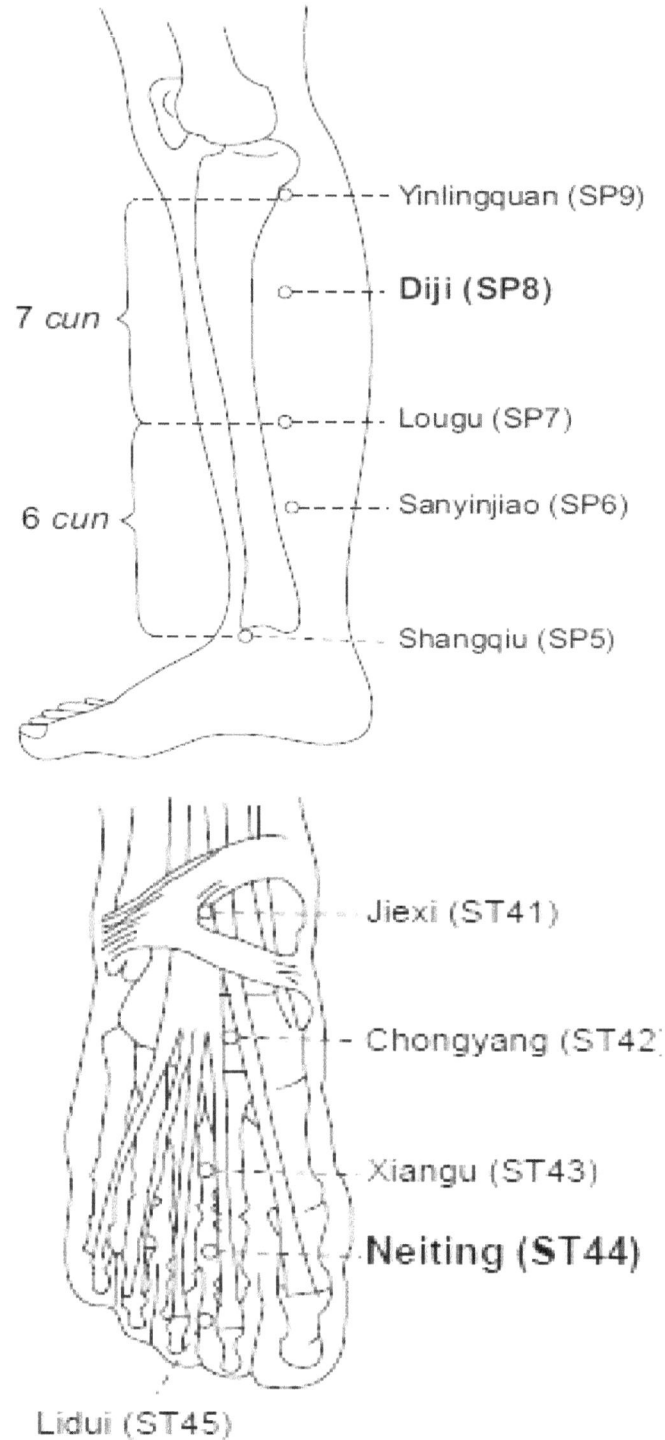

Hematemesis and/or Epistaxis during Menstruation

Taichong (LR3)–Neiting (ST44)

Electro-acupuncture is performed. Insert 40-mm needles into Taichong (LR3) and 25-mm needles into Neiting (ST44). After achieving a needle pricking sensation, connect the needles with an electro-acupuncture machine. Leave the needles in place for 30 min.

We have used this method for successfully treating hematemesis and/or epistaxis during menstruation in one case. This is for your reference.

Hematemesis and/or epistaxis during menstruation is caused by heat in the blood, reversed Qi flow, and hyperactivity of fire in the liver and stomach. It can also be caused by Yin deficiency, lung dryness, and bleeding due to heat. Therefore, it is treated according to the theory of lowering adverse, such as clearing heat, descending adverse Qi, and guiding the blood to flow downward. The Taichong (LR3) is the Shu-Stream point of the liver meridian, whereas The Neiting (ST44) is the Xing-Spring point. Treatment using a combination of these points can be used to suppress liver hyperactivity, clear stomach fire, regulate Qi and blood flow, clear excessive heat, and lower adverse Qi.

Hematemesis and/or Epistaxis during Menstruation

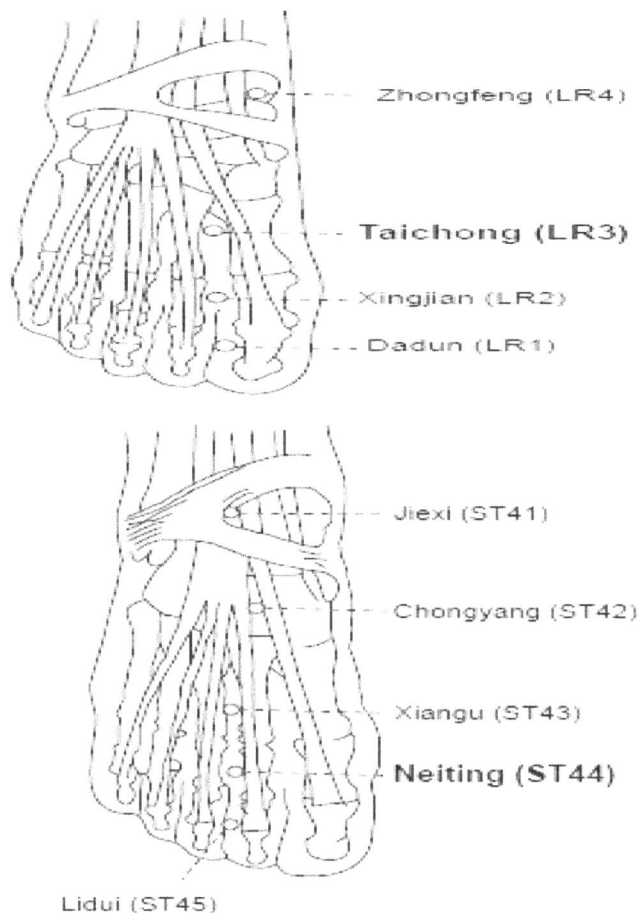

Zhongfeng (LR4)

Taichong (LR3)

Xingjian (LR2)

Dadun (LR1)

Jiexi (ST41)

Chongyang (ST42)

Xiangu (ST43)

Neiting (ST44)

Lidui (ST45)

Morbid Vaginal Discharge

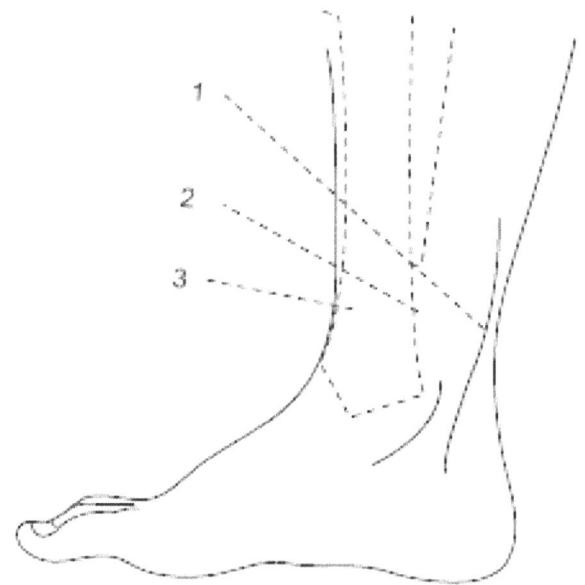

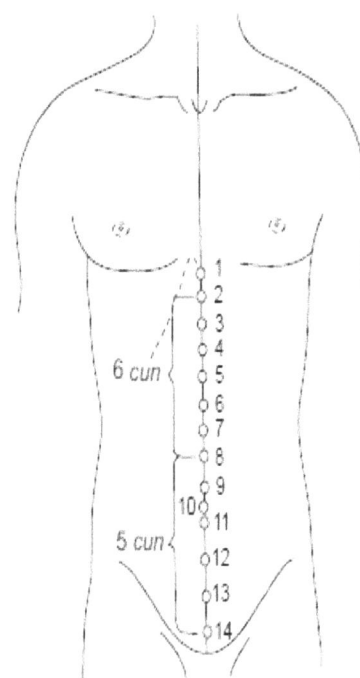

Morbid vaginal discharge refers to an increased amount or a discoloration of vaginal discharge. It is usually caused by an insecurity of the Conception Vessel, downward diffusing dampness, damage of the spleen and stomach due to diet or overwork, heat transformation from dampness stagnation, or dampness-heat diffusion downward.

Xiaerdian (wrist-ankle point)–Qugu (CV2)

Qugu (CV2): Located on the midline of the lower abdomen at the midpoint of the superior edge of the pubic symphysis.

Xiaerdian (wrist-ankle point): Located 3 fingers above the top of the medial malleolus on the posterior border of the tibia.

Acupuncture is performed. Insert a needle perpendicularly into the Qugu (CV2) at 2.5–3 *cun* deep, radiating the needle pricking sensation to the vagina. Two additional needles are inserted into the Xiaerdian at 1.4 *cun* deep. Leave the needles in place for 20–30 min.

Morbid Vaginal Discharge

1. Jiuwei (CV15)
2. Juque (CV14)
3. Shangwan (CV13)
4. Zhongwan (CV12)
5. Jianli (CV11)
6. Xiawan (CV10)
7. Shuifen (CV9)
8. Shenque (CV8)
9. Yinjiao (CV7)
10. Qihai (CV6)
11. Shimen (CV5)
12. Guanyuan (CV4)
13. Zhongji (CV3)
14. Qugu (CV2)

Uterine Prolapse

Uterine Prolapse

Uterine prolapse refers to the downward movement of the uterus from its normal position along the vagina. Common symptoms include sensation of heaviness on the lower abdomen, low back pain, trouble in urinating, incontinence, frequent urination, and uterine prolapse from the vagina.

Zhaohai (KI6)–Taichong (LR3)

Acupuncture is performed. Ask the patient to lie on her back. After sterilization, insert 0.38 * 25-mm needles into the points, performing the uniform reinforcing–reducing needle technique.

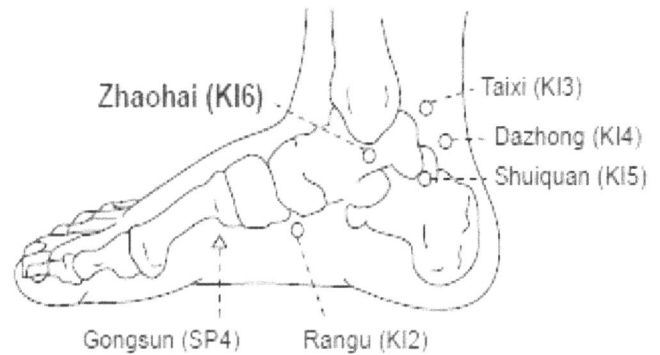

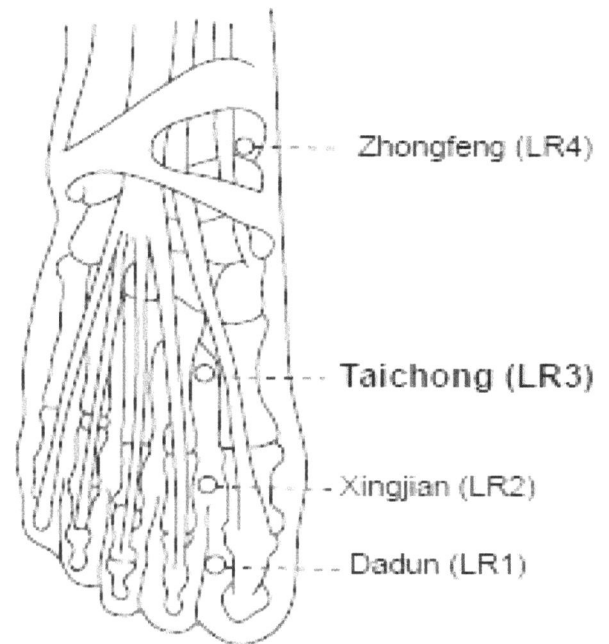

137

Perimenopausal Syndrome

Dazhong (KI4)–Taixi (KI3)

Acupuncture is performed. After sterilization, insert 40-mm into the Dazhong (KI4). After achieving the needle pricking sensation, perform the reducing needle technique. Then, insert40-mm needles into the Taixi (KI3), performing the reinforcing needle technique. Manipulate the needles once every 5 min and leave the needles in place for 20 min.

Case: Ms. Huang, a 49-year-old housewife, complained of vexation, heat in the hands and feet, chest tightness, insomnia, short of breath, and bad temper. We diagnosed her with perimenopausal syndrome and treated her with this method combined with the herbal medicine Jiawei Xiaoyao Powder. After two series of treatments (approximately 10 times), the symptoms disappeared completely.

Perimenopausal Syndrome

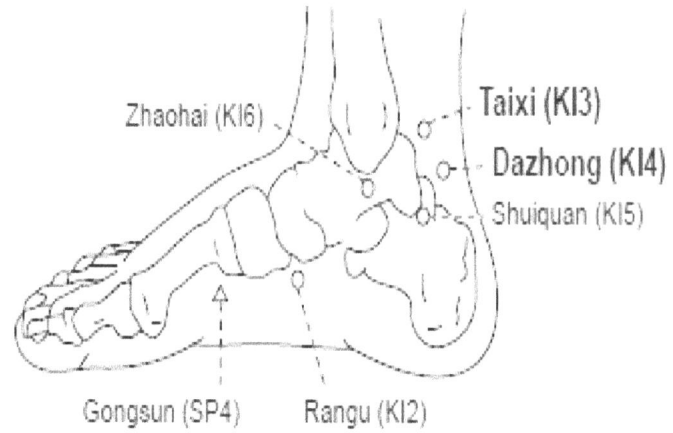

Infertility

Infertility

Guilai (ST29)–Sanyinjiao (SP6)

Acupuncture is performed. Insert 50-mm needles into the Guilai (ST29). Then, insert the needles obliquely into the Sanyinjiao (SP6) at 1.5 *cun* deep. The needle pricking sensation should radiate upward to the lower abdomen, along the inner side of leg. Leave the needles in place for 30 min.

Infertility in women is usually caused by essence and blood deficiency or by deficient uterine cold. Infertility can cause depression, liver stagnation, and blood deficiency. Therefore, the treatment should focus on reducing the excess and reinforcing the deficiency.

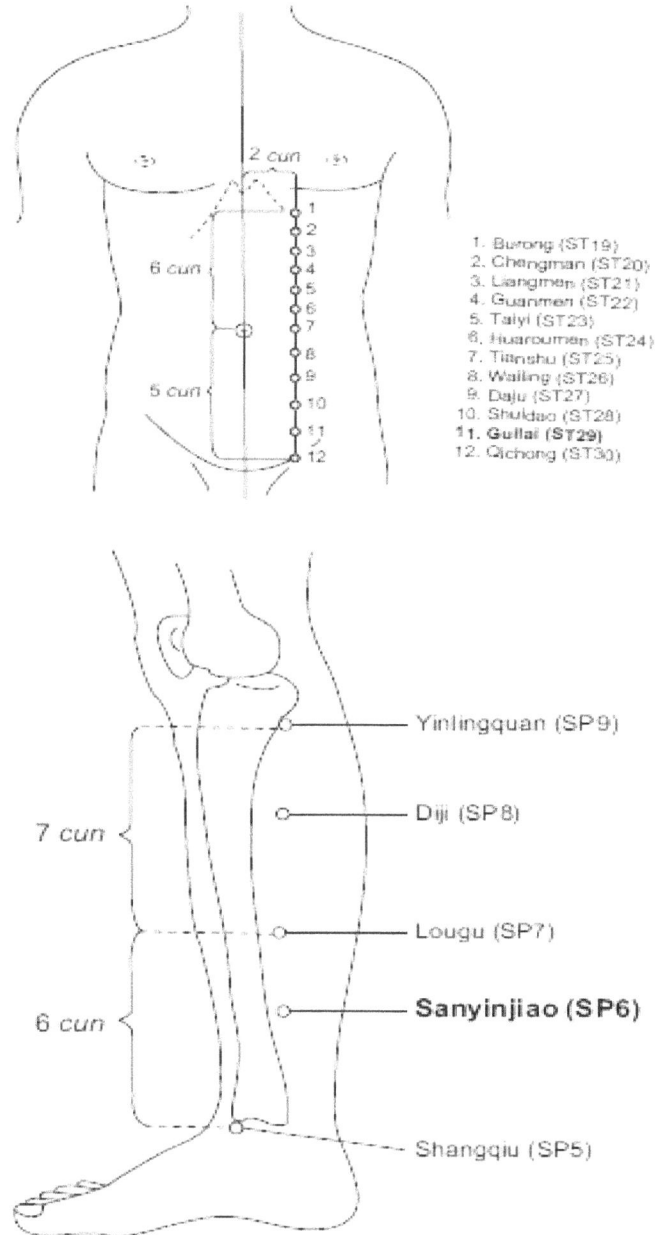

1. Burong (ST19)
2. Chengman (ST20)
3. Liangmen (ST21)
4. Guanmen (ST22)
5. Taiyi (ST23)
6. Huaroumen (ST24)
7. Tianshu (ST25)
8. Wailing (ST26)
9. Daju (ST27)
10. Shuidao (ST28)
11. Guilai (ST29)
12. Qichong (ST30)

Yinlingquan (SP9)

Diji (SP8)

Lougu (SP7)

Sanyinjiao (SP6)

Shangqiu (SP5)

Formula One: Zhiyin (BL67)–Sanyinjiao (SP6)

Method One: Acupuncture is performed. Insert the needles into the Zhiyin (BL67) at 0.3 *cun* deep. Insert the needles slightly upward into the Sanyinjiao (SP6) with the right hand at 0.8–1 *cun* deep. Press the Sanyinjiao (SP6) beneath the inserted needles with the left hand. The needle pricking sensation should radiate upward along the meridian. Leave the needles in place for 20 min, manipulating the needles once every 10 min.

Method Two: Moxibustion is performed. Ask the patient to sit. Perform sparrow-pecking moxibustion on the Zhiyin (BL67) for approximately 10 min until the skin turns red. Then, perform moxibustion on the Sanyinjiao (SP6). Movement of the abdominal wall can be observed. Perform this therapy until examination reveals a normal fetal position.

Formula Two: Fuke (11.24)–Jiemei (88.04, 88.05, and 88.06)

Acupuncture is performed. Insert the needles perpendicularly into the points. Select the Fuke (11.24) with a single hand and insert 100-mm needles into the Jiemei (88.04, 88.05, and 88.06).

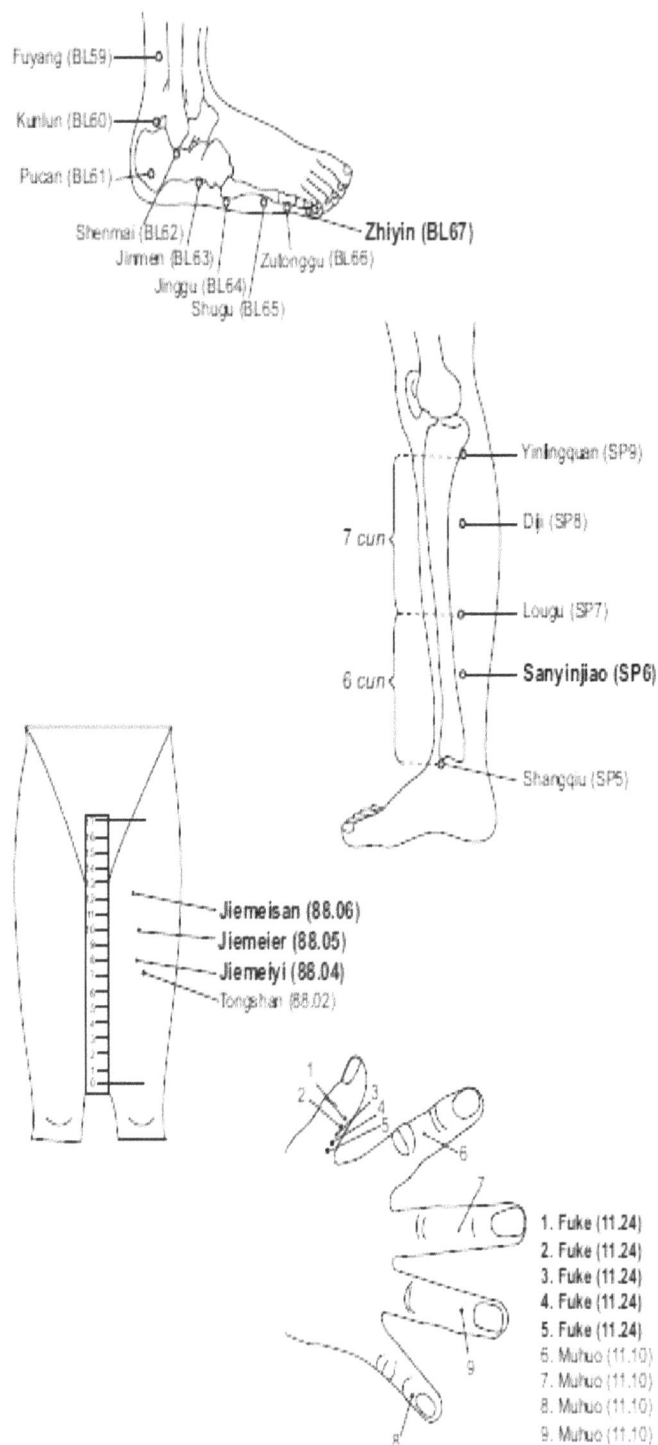

Hyperemesis Gravidarum

Hyperemesis Gravidarum

Taiyuan (LU9)–Cuanzhu (BL2)

Acupuncture is performed. Insert needles into the Taiyuan (LU9) on both sides, with the tips toward the Neiguan (PC6). Insert needles into the Cuanzhu (BL2) on both sides, with the tips toward Yintang. It is better to ask the patient to lie down when performing this therapy. Because pregnant women may have lower blood pressure, they tend to get sick when undergoing acupuncture.

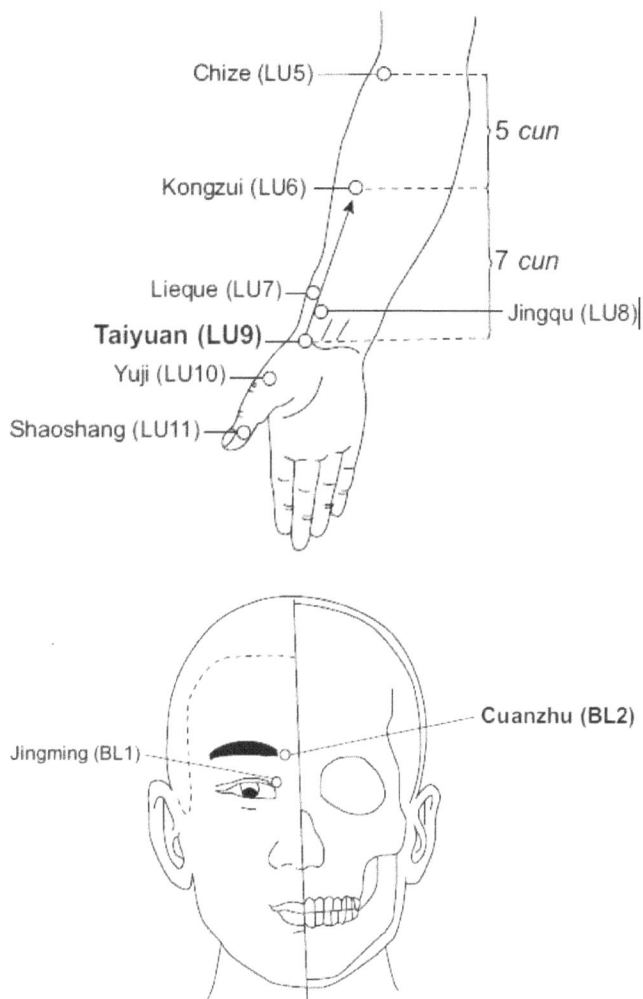

Post-term Pregnancy

Hegu (LI4)–Sanyinjiao (SP6)

Electro-acupuncture is performed. Insert the needles into the Hegu (LI4) and Sanyinjiao (SP6) and once the needle pricking sensation is achieved, connect the needles with the electro-acupuncture machine. Stimulation with dilatational wave should be performed for 20 min. Then, switch to the continuous wave for 10 min. Leave the needles in place for 30 min. The electric current intensity should be within the patient's tolerance range. This treatment should be performed once daily for 3 days.

Post-term pregnancy is usually caused by a Yang deficiency, Yin excess, or lack of activity during pregnancy. Both Hegu (LI4) and Sanyinjiao (SP6) are effective in hastening parturition by enhancing uterine contraction. Acupuncture on a combination of these two points can be used for reinforcing blood, regulating Qi, and hastening parturition. Electro-acupuncture can intensify stimulation and enhance uterine contraction.

Post-term Pregnancy

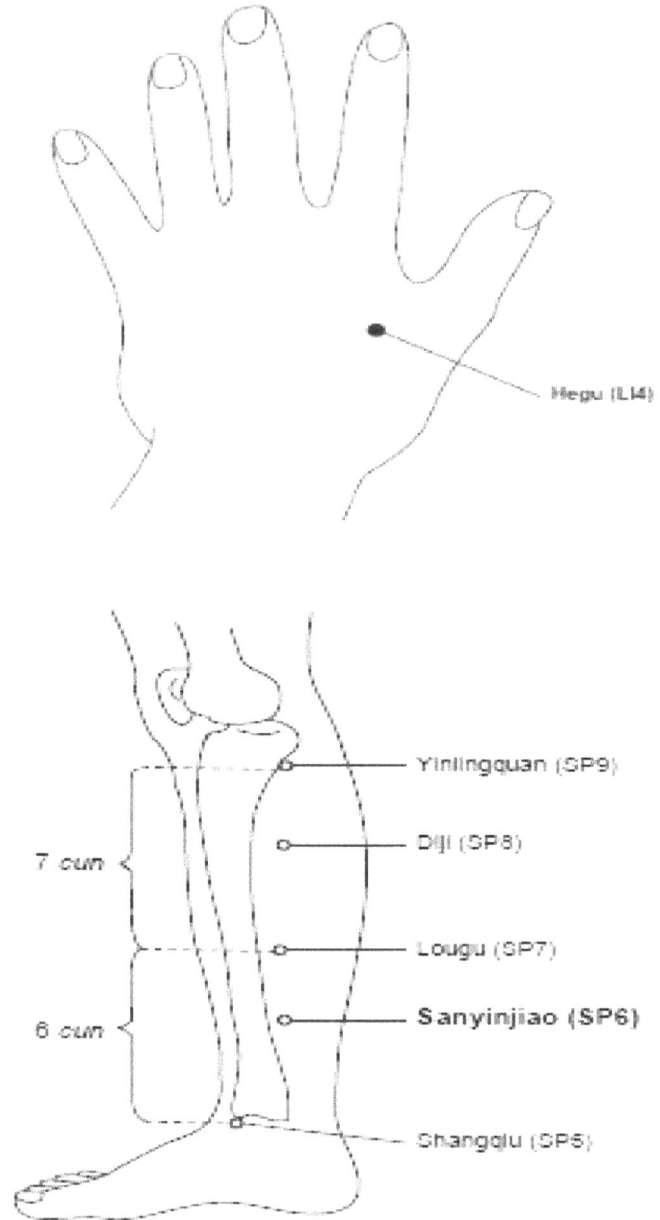

Abdominal Pain after Induction of Labor

Xuehai (SP10)–Sanyinjiao (SP6)

Acupuncture is performed. Ask the patient to lie on her back. Insert0.25 *-50 mm needles into the points quickly, then slowly remove the needles. Perform moderate stimulation without leaving the needles in place.

According to the theory of traditional Chinese medicine, abdominal pain after induction of labor is caused by blood deficiency and stagnation and by disharmony of Qi and blood. Pain can be accompanied by hemorrhage or lochioschesis. The hemorrhage may often disappear without treatment, whereas lochioschesis can be effectively treated with this method. The Sanyinjiao (SP6) is a convergence of the three-foot Yin meridians, which can be used for regulating Qi and the blood. The Xuehai (SP10) is a point on the spleen meridian. Because the spleen controls the blood, acupuncture on the Xuehai (SP10) can activate blood, dissipate stasis, and reinforce deficiency and Qi.

Abdominal Pain after Induction of Labor

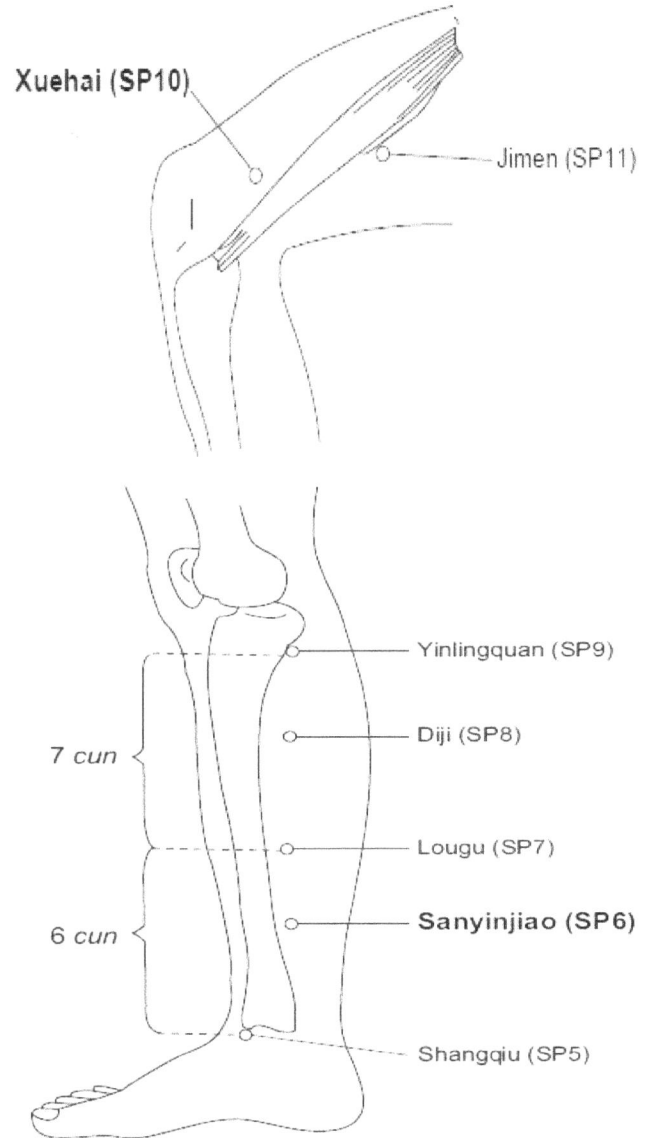

143

Terminating Lactation

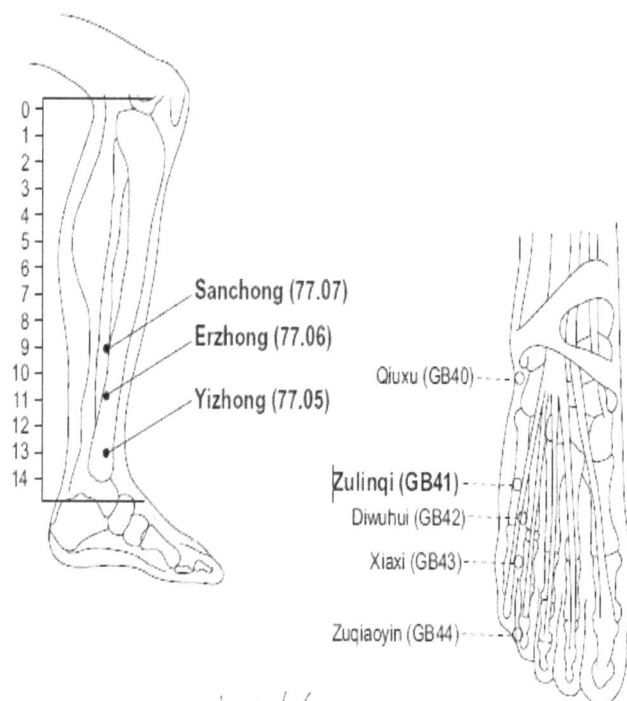

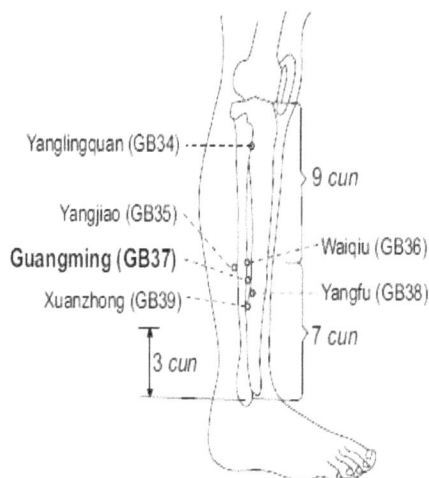

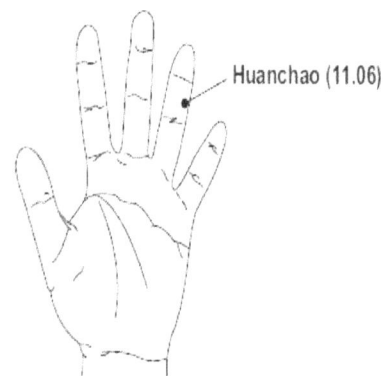

Formula One: Guangming (GB37)–Zulinqi (GB41)

Acupuncture is performed. Ask the patient to lie on her back. After sterilization, insert 0.27–0.32-mm needles into the points, performing the lifting and thrusting needle technique. Leave the needles in place for 20 min. Perform the treatment once a day. Usually, lactation can be terminated after one or two treatments.

Formula Two: Huanchao (11.06)–Sanchong (77.05, 77.06, 77.07)

Acupuncture is performed. Insert the needles perpendicularly into the points, performing the needle control technique. When inserting needles into Sanchong (77.05, 77.06, 77.07), the Daoma technique should be used.

Terminating Lactation

Chapter Eight

Miscellaneous Diseases

Quit Smoking

Only few individuals in Taiwan desire to quit smoking. However, in Europe and America, many individuals are willing to quit smoking. Because insurance payments in several developed countries are extremely high, numerous insurance companies will survey whether an applicant smokes. Therefore, individuals in those countries pay more attention in keeping themselves healthy.

Tianwei–Hegu (LI4)

Tianwei: An extra point located at the midpoint of the line between the Yangxi (LI5) and Lieque (LU7).

Combination treatment of acupuncture and topical application is performed. The same amount of ding xiang (clove) and rougui (cassia bark) is ground into a fine powder. The powder is mixed with water, and monosodium glutamate is added to the mixture. The medicine is mixed with warm water to keep it warm. Approximately 1 g of the medicine is used to make one medicine cake. The medicine cake is then placed on the point after performing acupuncture twice every day. Normally, the patient can quit smoking after undergoing the treatment for 1 week.

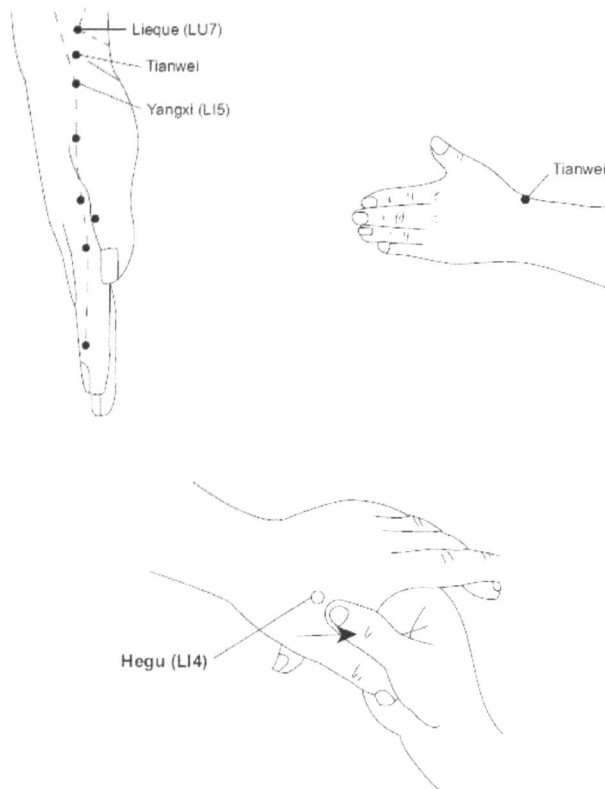

Lieque (LU7)
Tianwei
Yangxi (LI5)
Tianwei
Hegu (LI4)

Abstaining from Alcohol

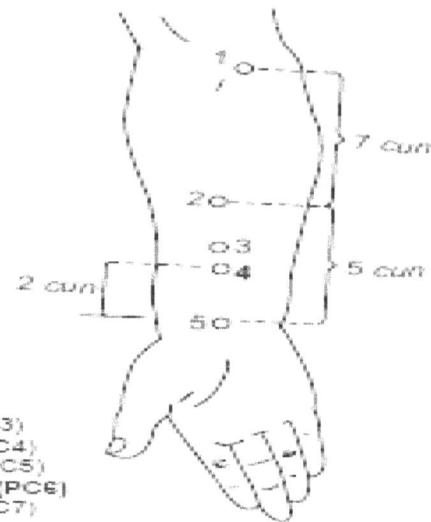

Abstaining from Alcohol

Neiguan (PC6)–Lieque (LU7)

Acupuncture is performed. Insert 40-mm needles perpendicularly into the Neiguan (PC) at 1 *cun* deep. Insert the needles obliquely into the Lieque (LU7) just under the skin. Perform the reducing needle technique. Leave the needles in place for 30 min once every day.

After treatment once or twice with this method, a patient can usually abstain from drinking alcohol or reduce the amount of drinking.

Neiguan (PC6) is a point on the pericardium meridian and is one of the eight confluence points. It can be used for treating diseases of stomach, heart, and chest. It also has the function of tranquillization. Lieque (LU7) is the Luo point of the lung meridian. This point is close to the large intestine meridian, and it connects with the conception vessel. Patients who are alcoholic are usually considered to have disorders of the lung, stomach, and large intestine. Therefore, these two points are selected.

1. Quze (PC3)
2. Ximen (PC4)
3. Jianshi (PC5)
4. Neiguan (PC6)
5. Daling (PC7)

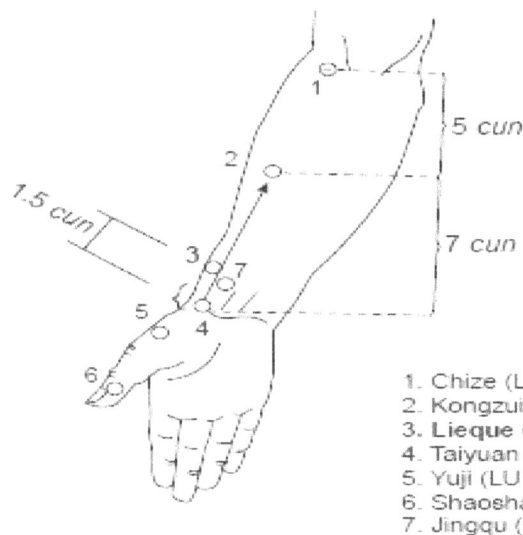

1. Chize (LU5)
2. Kongzui (LU6)
3. Lieque (LU7)
4. Taiyuan (LU9)
5. Yuji (LU10)
6. Shaoshang (LU11)
7. Jingqu (LU8)

Hegu (LI4)–Neiguan (PC6)

Acupuncture is performed. Insert 40-mm needles into the Hegu (LI4), with the tips of the points positioned toward the Houxi (SI3). Perform the reducing needle technique with lifting and thrusting. Insert 40-mm needles into the Neiguan (PC6), with the tips of the points positioned toward the Waiguan (TE5). Perform the reducing needle technique with twisting and twirling. After achieving the needle pricking sensation, leave the needles in place for 30 min.

Hegu (LI4) is the Yuan-source point or a point on the large intestine meridian, which is a Yangming meridian. The stomach meridian is also a Yangming meridian. Meridians with the same characteristics can be used together as Qi on different pathways will interact with each other. Therefore, stimulation on the Hegu (LI4) can clear fire of the stomach, dispel wind, resolve superficial pathogens, and activate collaterals. Performing the reducing needle technique on the Neiguan (PC6) can regulate Qi, harmonize the stomach, and relieve chest tightness. Therefore, these two points can be used together for eliminating the effects of alcohol.

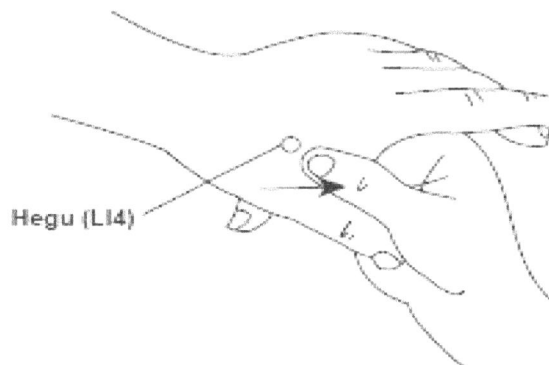

Hegu (LI4)

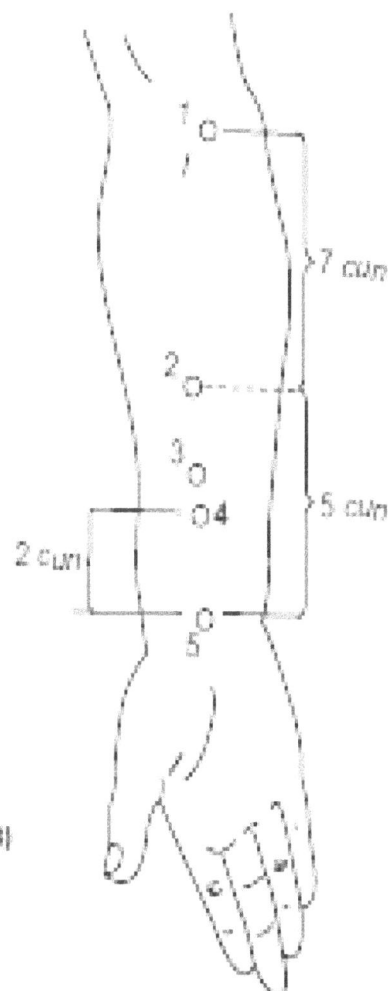

7 cun

5 cun

2 cun

1. Quze (PC3)
2. Ximen (PC4)
3. Jianshi (PC5)
4. Neiguan (PC6)
5. Daling (PC7)

Losing Weight

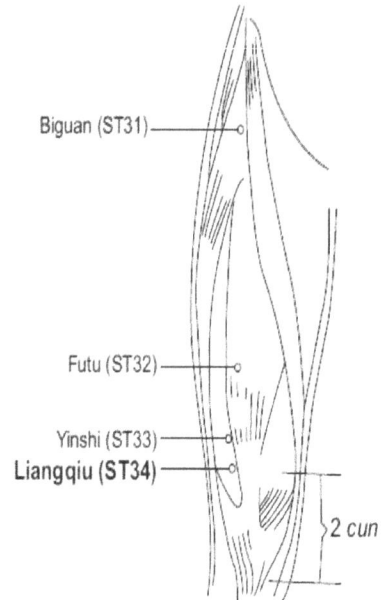

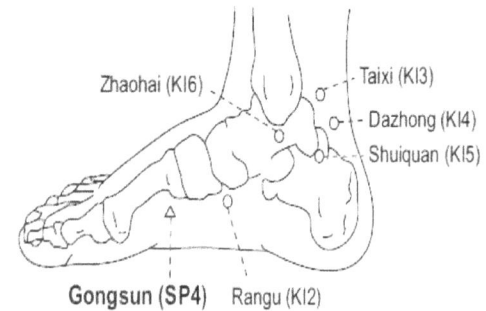

Losing Weight

Liangqiu (ST34)–Gongsun (SP4)

Electroacupuncture is performed. Insert the needles into the points. Connect the needle handles with the electro-acupuncture machine. Use discontinuous wave to perform a strong stimulation. After treatment for 20 min, remove the needles. Perform intradermal needle therapy on these points. Ask the patient to press the points 3–4 times when he/she feels hungry or 10 min before meals. Perform the therapy for 3 days. Then, pause for 1 week before starting another session of treatment for 3 days.

Quit Masturbation

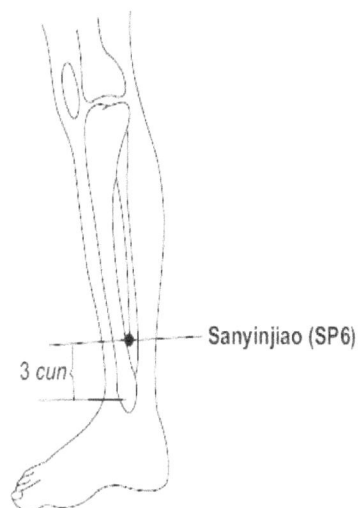

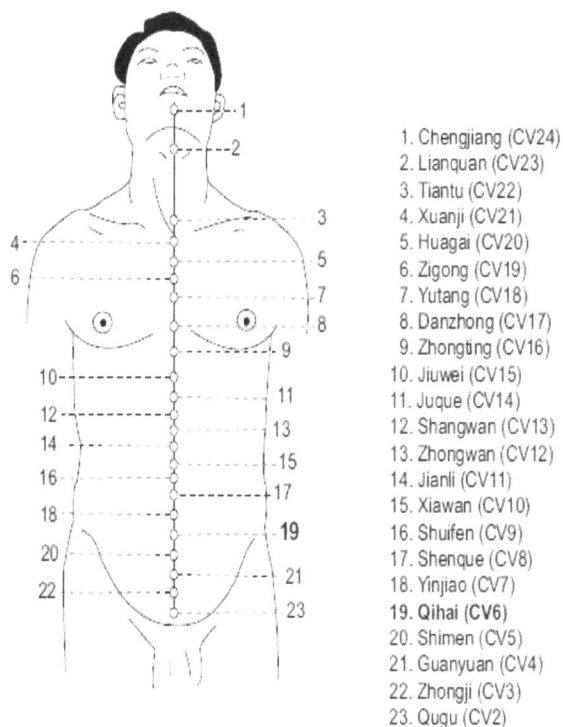

Quit Masturbation

Qihai (CV6)–Sanyingjiao (SP6)

Acupuncture is performed. Insert a needle horizontally into the Qihai (CV6), with the tip of the needle positioned toward the Shenque (CV8). Perform the reducing needle technique with twisting and twirling. Insert 40-mm needles into the Sanyinjiao (SP6) at 1.2 *cun* deep, and then, perform the reducing needle technique with lifting and thrusting. The needle pricking sensation should radiate upward. After achieving the needle pricking sensation, leave the needles in place for 30 min. Perform the treatment once every other day.

3 cun — Sanyinjiao (SP6)

1. Chengjiang (CV24)
2. Lianquan (CV23)
3. Tiantu (CV22)
4. Xuanji (CV21)
5. Huagai (CV20)
6. Zigong (CV19)
7. Yutang (CV18)
8. Danzhong (CV17)
9. Zhongting (CV16)
10. Jiuwei (CV15)
11. Juque (CV14)
12. Shangwan (CV13)
13. Zhongwan (CV12)
14. Jianli (CV11)
15. Xiawan (CV10)
16. Shuifen (CV9)
17. Shenque (CV8)
18. Yinjiao (CV7)
19. **Qihai (CV6)**
20. Shimen (CV5)
21. Guanyuan (CV4)
22. Zhongji (CV3)
23. Qugu (CV2)

Motion Sickness

Motion Sickness

Eryuan–Shenque (CV8)

Stick seed (stainless steel ear pellets) at the points before getting aboard. Usually, immediate effectiveness can be achieved. For patients who are experiencing motion sickness for a long time, the points can be pressed with the hand at ordinary times. The points are effective in regulating disorder of the balance system in the internal ear.

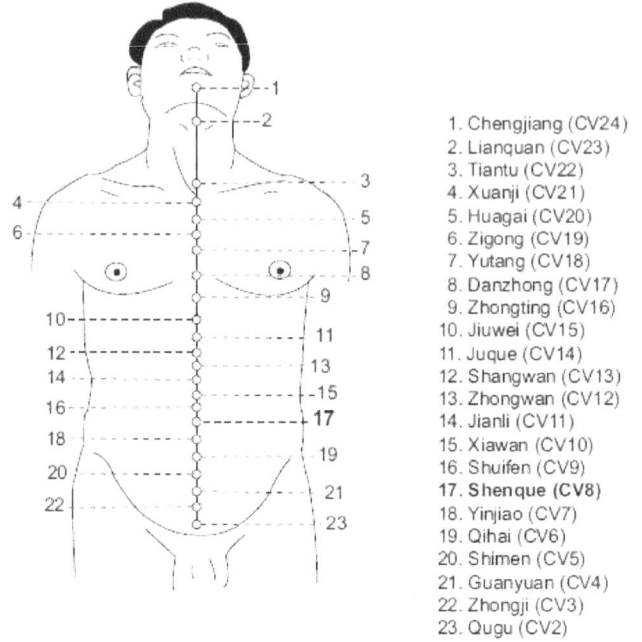

1. Chengjiang (CV24)
2. Lianquan (CV23)
3. Tiantu (CV22)
4. Xuanji (CV21)
5. Huagai (CV20)
6. Zigong (CV19)
7. Yutang (CV18)
8. Danzhong (CV17)
9. Zhongting (CV16)
10. Jiuwei (CV15)
11. Juque (CV14)
12. Shangwan (CV13)
13. Zhongwan (CV12)
14. Jianli (CV11)
15. Xiawan (CV10)
16. Shuifen (CV9)
17. **Shenque (CV8)**
18. Yinjiao (CV7)
19. Qihai (CV6)
20. Shimen (CV5)
21. Guanyuan (CV4)
22. Zhongji (CV3)
23. Qugu (CV2)

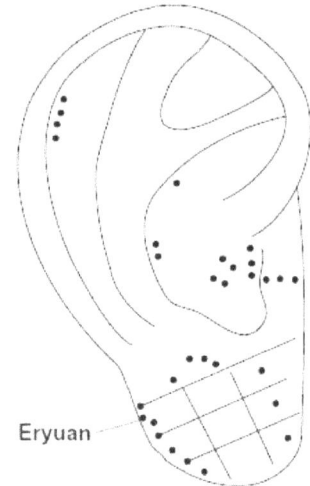

Eryuan

Postoperative Pain

Postoperative Pain

Daling (PC7)–Fengshi (GB31)

Acupuncture is performed. Insert the needles into the points on both sides, with no specific needle technique. When inserting the needles into the Daling (PC7), it is better to ask the patient to hold his/her breath before insertion. Leave the needles in place for 20–30 min. Manipulate the needles for 5 more min and then remove them.

Usually, >50% of the pain can be relieved after one treatment.

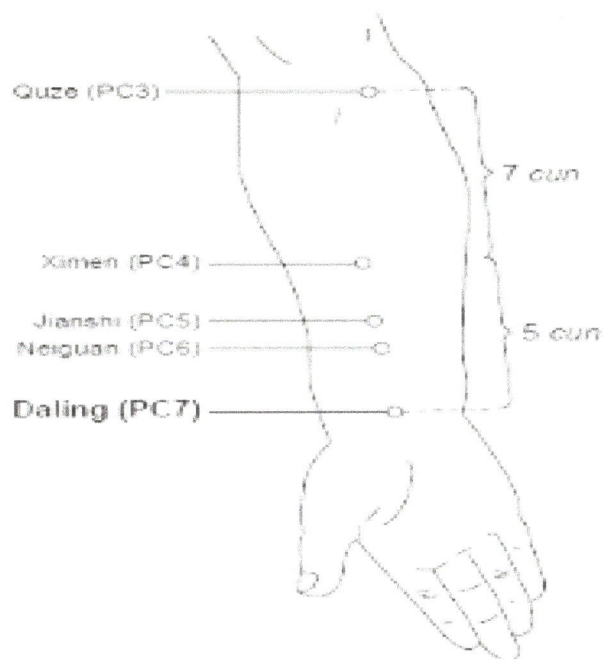

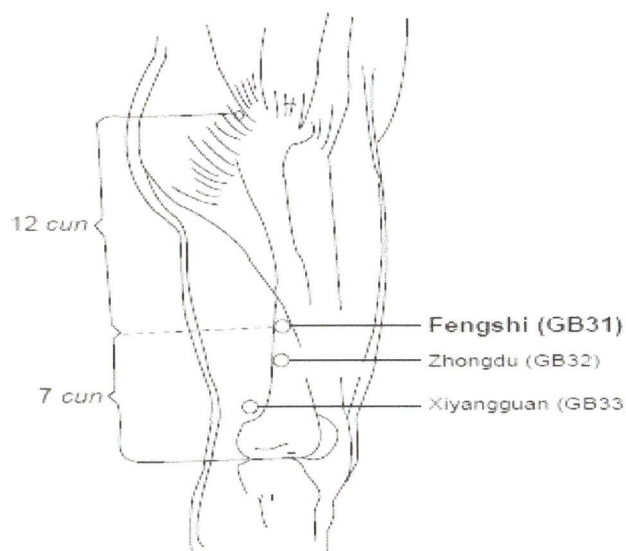

Stress

Stress

Zhenjing (1010.08)–Huoying (66.03)

Acupuncture is performed. Insert the needles into the Zhenjing (1010.08) and Huoying (66.03) at 3–5 *fen* deep, without performing the needle technique. Ask the patient to lie on his/her back for 20–30 min. Subsequently, remove the needles.

In practice, patients treated with this method can feel less stress than before. Combine the therapy with herbal medicine. Normally, the patients can be cured after 1–2 treatments.

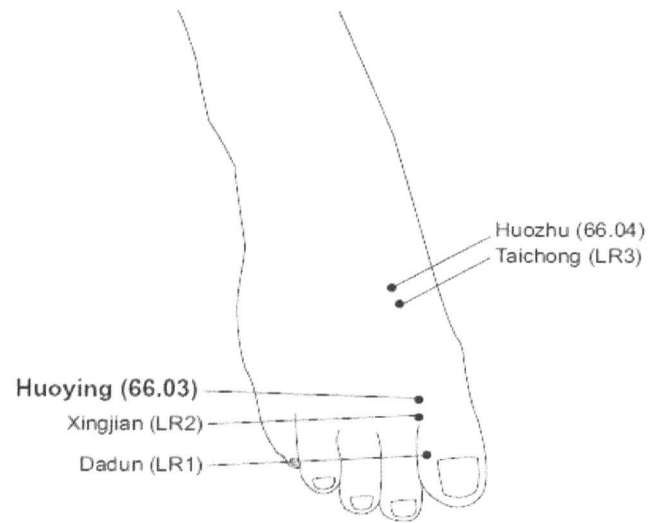

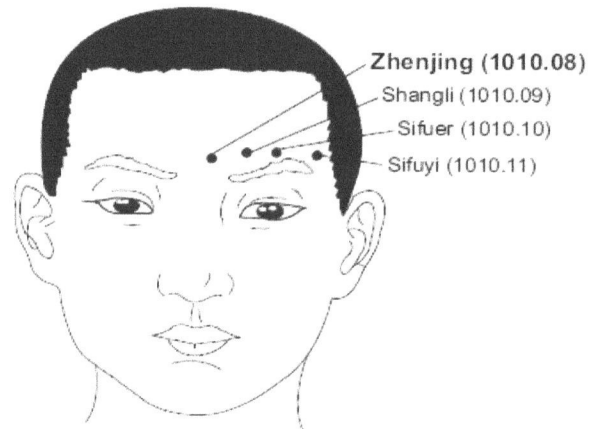

Precious pictures of Mr. Tung's extraordinary points by Dr. Chien

Dr. Tung Chingchang and Dr. Lin Chixian are also teachers of Dr. Chien. Both Dr Tung and Lin are from Shandong, China and have been friends for many years. When Master Tung visited California for a meeting, he was treated by Dr. Lin Chixian and he lodged at his home in New Port Beach. Dr. Lin Chixian became famous in California's South Bay area and even the Mayor of New Port Beach came to see him. For Master Tung, Lin Chixian was not only a friend from his province but also a partner for learning medical skills. Master Tung also used his time in California to discuss teaching acupuncture and moxibustion medical expertise and diagnosis with Professor Chixian. After the death of Master Tung, Dr. Lin Chixian took time to attend the funeral and then returned to California to pass on his medical skills to his disciple, Dr. Chien.

Doctor Calvin Chien is the only practitioner in the world who can perform palmar diagnosis as Mr. Tung's disciple and is the only doctor with 30 years of actual clinical experience with Mr. Tung's extraordinary points.

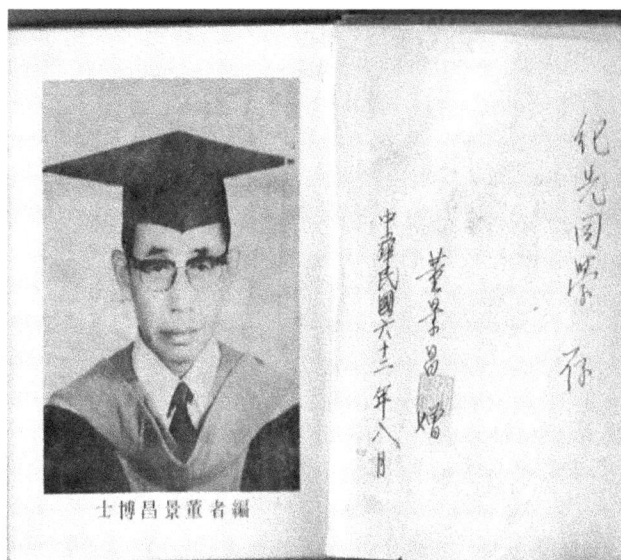

Picture 1:

Description: In 1973, Master Tung presented his signature and inscription to Dr. Lin on the back cover of "Mr. Tung's school of Acupuncture and Moxibustion channels and extraordinary points." The difference from donations to other disciples of Mr. Tung is that Mr. Tung's inscription here states "Lin Chixian's schoolmate," which makes it obvious that he treated his fellow countryman as a peer (provided by Dr. Calvin).

Inscription: From Right to Left

The first line of the text is "For Chixian's students," the second line is "Tung Chingchang's present," and the third line is "photo of the Republic of China in August, 73"

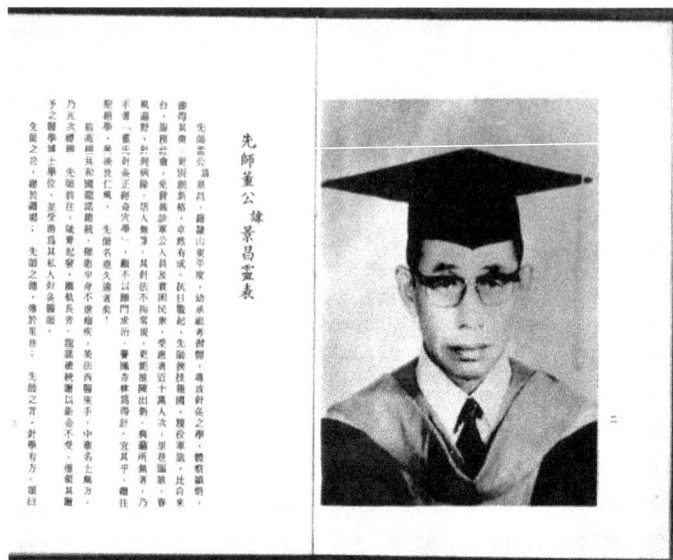

Picture 2 From Left to Right

Inscription: Acupuncture and moxibustion clinical experience of Mr. Tung's five generations of ancestors

Dr. Lin Chixian, June, 1984

Picture 3

Master Tung Chingchang's portrait and biography from the book "Mr. Tung's acupuncture and moxibustion" (provided by Dr. Calvin).

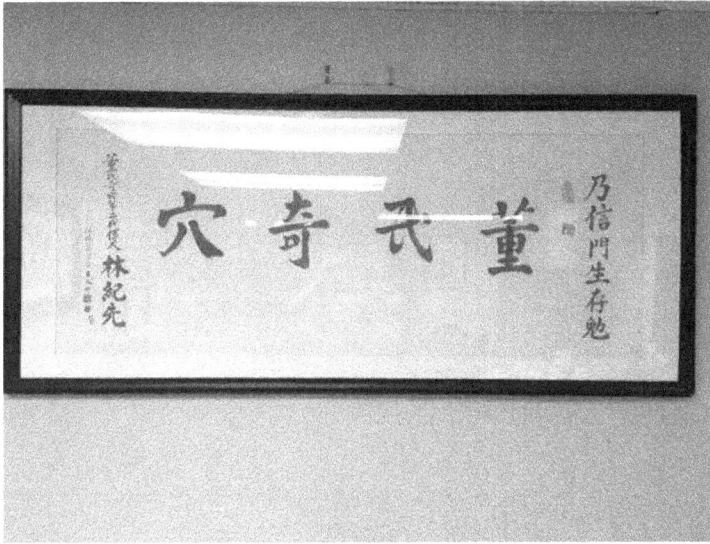

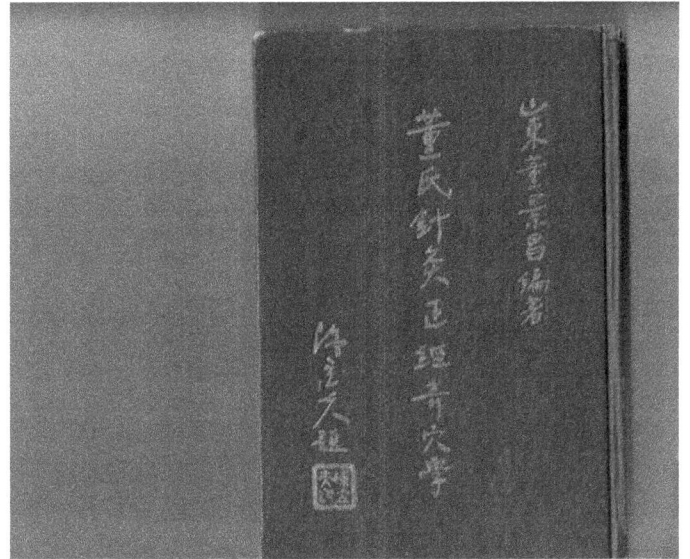

Picture 4

Description: The memorial plague given by Dr. Lin to Dr. Calvin

Inscription : From Right to Left Naisin student remembering Tung's extraordinary points Lin Chixian, the second generation of disciple of Mr. Tung's extraordinary points Inscribed by Wang Chengzhong at the eight hundred bridge, Liuhe, Jiangsu

Picture 5

Description: : Mr. Tung presented Dr. Lin with the book "Mr. Tung's school of Acupuncture and Moxibustion orthodox channels and extraordinary points" and Lin Chixian later passed it on to Dr. Calvin Chien (provided by Dr. Calvin).

Inscription: From Right to Left

Tung Chingchang edited in Shandong Mr. Tung's acupuncture and moxibustion Reviewed by Chen Lifu

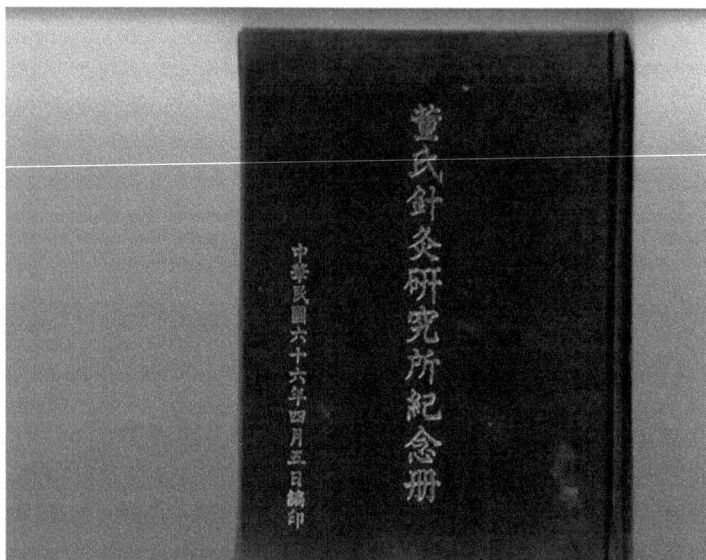

Picture 6

Description: "Mr. Tung's commemorative album of the institute of acupuncture and moxibustion." These are commemorative works published by Tung's students after his death. They are not issued in the market (provided by Dr. Calvin).

Inscription: From Right to Left

Mr. Tung's Acupuncture Research Institute Published on April 5, 1966

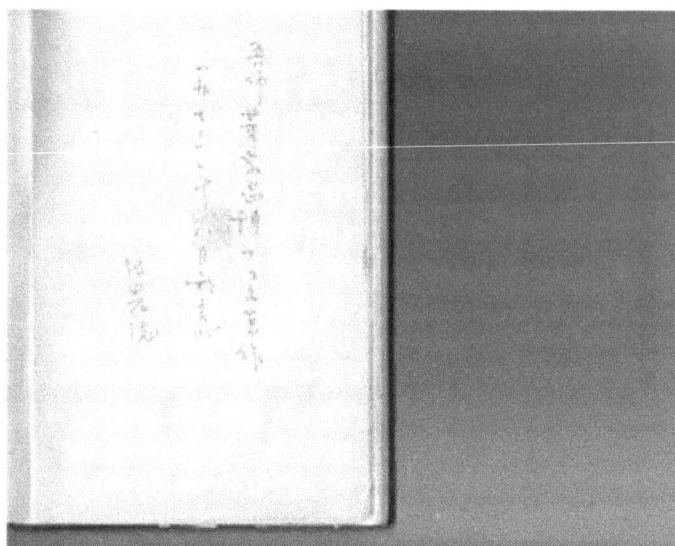

Picture 7

Inscription: From Right to Lefts

The masterpiece of my teacher, Dr. Tung Chingchang August 1973 in Taipei,

Lin Chixian